ZEN
CAREGIVING

Praise for *Zen Caregiving*

"Caregivers like Roy Remer are the unsung heroes and heroines of our world. Roy's many years volunteering in a hospice setting translate to pages suffused with wisdom, love, and immensely practical advice for the caregiver. A gem of a book!"

— **Abraham Verghese, MD**, author of *Cutting for Stone* and *The Covenant of Water* and director of the PRESENCE Center, Stanford School of Medicine

"I often teach that Zen is really a code word for 'human.' Zen caregiving, or human caregiving, is a simple and profound shift of awareness, from turning away to turning toward impermanence and the fact that we are all caregivers and will all be care receivers. This is a beautiful and practical guide for being transformed as we open our hearts to what matters most."

— **Marc Lesser**, author of *Seven Practices of a Mindful Leader: Lessons from Google and a Zen Monastery Kitchen*

"*Zen Caregiving* isn't another manual — it's a friend sitting beside you, acknowledging that caregiving cracks you open. Each chapter offers concrete meditation exercises and Gathas — portable verses for difficult moments — designed to fit caregivers' limited time. The book beautifully prompts self-reflection, inviting readers to examine their experiences with compassion while normalizing struggles. From reading it, you understand that self-care isn't indulgent but essential to sustainable caregiving. Whether you're beginning your journey or feeling burned-out, *Zen Caregiving* offers a transformative path forward for one of life's most meaningful experiences."

— **BJ Miller, MD**, coauthor of *A Beginner's Guide to the End*

"*Zen Caregiving* is a book that understands something modern medicine often forgets: Caring is not only about doing, but about being. Roy Remer writes about the quality of presence that sustains every technical act. And that changes everything. There is a rare honesty in this work. It does not promise constant lightness, nor does it romanticize caregiving. It names fatigue, silent resentment, and moral exhaustion without apology. Precisely because of that, it presents self-compassion not as a luxury, but as a prerequisite for genuine compassion."

— **Dr. Ana Claudia Quintana Arantes**, author of *Death Is a Day Worth Living*

"In this beautiful, moving, and life-changing book, Roy Remer's writing embodies the beautiful qualities that he states are essential in mindful caregiving: kindness, empathy, and wisdom. Drawing on his vast experience of bearing witness bedside to the dying, Remer's book is a lucid, nuanced, yet practical companion for all caregivers, showing them how to walk that path with self-care, mindfulness, and compassion. I highly recommend that every caregiver read this book. It will be a great support for you and for those you care for."

— **Mark Coleman**, author of *Awake in the Wild* and *Make Peace with Your Mind*

"As a pastoral counselor, chaplain, and spiritual care scholar, I can attest to the fact that the ability to graciously face our shared existential situation is aided by what is in this book."

— **Pamela Ayo Yetunde, MA, ThD**, author of *Casting Indra's Net: Fostering Spiritual Kinship and Community*

ZEN CAREGIVING

How to Care for Yourself While Caring for Others

ROY REMER
Executive Director of Zen Caregiving Project

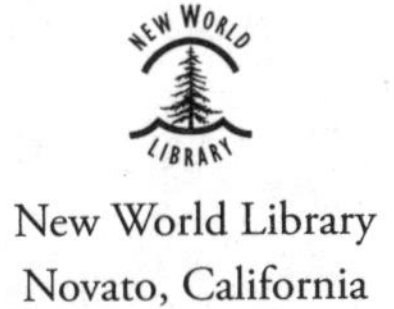

New World Library
Novato, California

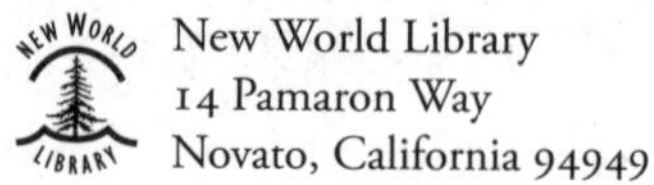

New World Library
14 Pamaron Way
Novato, California 94949

Text design by Tona Pearce Myers

Library of Congress Cataloging-in-Publication Data

Names: Remer, Roy, author
Title: Zen caregiving : how to care for yourself while caring for others / Roy Remer.
Description: Novato : New World Library, 2026. | Includes bibliographical references. | Summary: "From the executive director of Zen Caregiving Project comes a much-needed guide offering practical advice, emotional support, and spiritual solace for the millions of people around the world who must care for seriously ill family members or patients"-- Provided by publisher.
Identifiers: LCCN 2025053341 (print) | LCCN 2025053342 (ebook) | ISBN 9781608689538 paperback | ISBN 9781608689545 epub
Subjects: LCSH: Spiritual life--Zen Buddhism | Healing--Religious aspects--Buddhism | Mental health--Religious aspects--Buddhism
Classification: LCC BQ9288 .R46 2026 (print) | LCC BQ9288 (ebook) | DDC 294.3/444--dc23/eng/20260114
LC record available at https://lccn.loc.gov/2025053341
LC ebook record available at https://lccn.loc.gov/2025053342

First printing, April 2026
ISBN 978-1-60868-953-8
Ebook ISBN 978-1-60868-954-5
Printed in Canada

10 9 8 7 6 5 4 3 2 1

New World Library is committed to protecting our natural environment. This book is made of material from well-managed FSC®-certified forests and other controlled sources.

To my mother and father,
who taught me that caregiving is an expression of love.

Contents

Loss

Intimacy

Introduction

As it has for many others, my path to caregiving stemmed from a sense of responsibility, concern, and love. As a teenager I cherished time with my maternal grandmother, Bubbe Sylvia, who managed various chronic health conditions and needed help around her home and with errands. While I had moments of frustration and impatience as a young person, a deep desire to ease her life always lay beneath my occasional resistance.

In 1996, as Bubbe neared the end of her life, during a hospital visit she shared with me her readiness for death. I interpreted this as an invitation to connect with her in a new way. There was little she needed me to do physically; instead, I just sat by her side, listening and reassuring her of my love. At the time, I didn't fully grasp the vital role simple companionship plays in caregiving, nor did I realize how profoundly this experience, just weeks before her death, would transform my life.

As I navigated my grief following Bubbe's passing, I encountered two hospice volunteers. These kind and compassionate individuals worked with me at a small Buddhist publisher in Berkeley, California. I was deeply moved by their ability to create a safe space for me to express my grief. Patrick and Maria were comfortable witnessing my sadness and attentively listened to the broader story of my lifelong interest in loss and death. In time they guided me toward the Zen Hospice Project (ZHP) and its volunteer caregiver training program.

Through my experience as a volunteer caregiver, sitting at the bedsides of individuals facing serious and terminal illnesses, I discovered a new facet of myself and learned to forge deep connections with others through caregiving. I am incredibly fortunate to have had numerous generous teachers since my initial training. While some were ZHP volunteers or staff, the majority were individuals living their final days in hospice care. The profound gratitude I hold for those who shared their wisdom and welcomed me into the intimate experience of dying is a treasure that serves as the inspiration for this book.

Mindful Caregiving Education

In 2015 a colleague and I conceived of the Mindful Caregiving Education program (MCE). Initially, MCE repurposed much of the curriculum that had been developed for our well-known volunteer training. We were inspired to make available to caregivers the mindfulness-based approach to caregiving that had changed the lives of so many of our volunteers. After initially targeting caregivers who were caring for people at the end of life, we quickly realized the importance of pushing upstream to reach caregivers earlier. We discovered that caregivers who were supporting a loved one or friend at the end of their lives were often experiencing high levels of burden, even burnout. Promoting our courses to caregivers who were just getting started in the role was complementary to our end-of-life work.

At the time of MCE's inception, we looked around and found that although many wonderful caregiver-support programs focused on disease pathology or practical hands-on caregiving skills, none offered techniques for building emotional resilience the way our program did. This was the case for clinical and professional caregiver training programs, as well as for programs for family caregivers. We were also finding that most people who found themselves in the role of family caregiver were woefully unprepared for the responsibility. Even if they received training in how to assist with the activities of daily living, many reported not being ready for the emotional burden that family caregiving eventually presents.

Many of the caregivers we support speak of the significant sense of purpose and satisfaction that caregiving brings. However, some caregivers, typically those in the later stages of caregiving, share stories of the distress and overwhelm that come with caring for and witnessing a loved one struggling with advancing illness and disability. While long overdue, we are now beginning to see in media and politics recognition of the pervasiveness of family caregiving and the strain these undervalued caregivers experience.

Roselyn Carter summed up the human experience best when she said, "There are only four kinds of people in the world: those who have been caregivers, those who are currently caregivers, those who will be caregivers, and those who will need caregivers." The health and well-being of formal and informal caregivers, the backbone of our healthcare system, should be of concern to everyone.

Zen and No Zen

My goal in writing this book was to provide access to tools that support the emotional well-being of caregivers, the tools that changed my life. While the approach to care taught by the Zen Caregiving Project is often described as spiritual, rooted in a 2,500-hundred-year-old wisdom tradition, the practices included in this book fit perfectly in the secular modern world. Whatever your religious or spiritual background, you will likely recognize the fundamental human wisdom, common to all spiritual traditions, that has given rise to the practices shared in the pages that follow.

So what is Zen? Many teachers of Zen have written that if it is defined by words, it is not truly Zen. And while a rich body of Zen teachings has been passed down from teacher to teacher to student since the fifth century, the essence of Zen is experiential. To truly know Zen, you must practice it. Nonetheless, we point toward the meaning of the word *Zen* with words.

Often translated from the Japanese as a state of meditation or absorption, Zen is a clarity of mind accessed through direct experience of what is arising in the present moment. To me, Zen means experiencing life honestly and wholeheartedly in every waking moment, no matter what shows up in our path. This is not a book of Zen doctrine. This is an offering of teachings, perspectives, and practices inspired by the Zen philosophy I have been fortunate to study and work with for many years.

After I was introduced to Zen Buddhism in my early twenties, my understanding of the philosophy and practice was limited to what I acquired through reading books. When I lived in Japan as a college student, I witnessed the impact of Zen practice and philosophy on culture and lifestyle. However, it was not until I committed to a practice of meditation later in my life that I began to notice any change in my resilience and sense of well-being. It was through a committed practice of Zen meditation that I learned to maintain present-moment awareness, even off the meditation cushion.

The mindset that results from Zen practice can be described as mindful awareness, or mindfulness. Mindful awareness, or mindfulness, is sustained, nonjudgmental attention to what is happening right here, right now. Mindfulness is the attentive mind. It is being with things as they are, without turning away from or excluding anything from your direct experience. You do not have to be a student of Zen, or any form of Buddhism, to cultivate and benefit from mindfulness. This book will show you how to develop and sustain mindful awareness in the context of caregiving.

Benefits of Practicing

The more you practice mindfulness and mindful caregiving, the greater the impact you will notice. If you only read this book, there will be some benefits. However, if you work with the practices in each chapter, you will begin to notice a change in how you respond to the challenges you face in caregiving and in your life. Through practice, you will begin to notice that your sense of well-being is enhanced. Trust plays an important part in the process of becoming a more mindful caregiver, knowing that though change may not be immediate, it will come. And, like everyone else, you will falter from time to time, reacting to a situation unskillfully or losing contact with the experience of calm. Such missteps are human and crucial to your growth. When you stumble off the path, simply reorient yourself with kindness, and begin again. This is how you boost your resilience and well-being.

Working with the practices will be beneficial not only to you but to those you care for. The more resilient and stable you are, the better your care will be. You have likely heard it before, but it bears repeating: It is impossible to fully care for others if you are not caring for yourself. This is certainly true in the long term. Ultimately, this is a book about self-care. It demonstrates ways to tend to your own experience moment to moment while delivering care to others. I trust that whatever benefits you derive from reading this book will flow even beyond the current care relationship in your life.

Who Is a Caregiver?

I take a broad interpretation of the term *caregiver*. Being human means offering care. In a time when so many feel the lack of authentic community, caregiving reminds us that we are part of an interdependent network of relationships. We each depend on the support of others, and others depend on us. How you identify yourself in regard to the role of supporting others is ultimately up to you. However, whether you are paid to deliver care, or a daughter or son simply doing what a daughter or son does, or a partner showing up to meet the needs of your sweetie, or a parent taking responsibility for the well-being of your children, the people in your life will likely view you a caregiver.

When interacting with strangers in public, I remind myself that I have no idea what hardships they have experienced or are going through now. Though I don't always succeed, I try to engage anyone I encounter with attention and kindness as if I were their caregiver. Even when the person I meet appears to be different from me in regard to frame of mind, values, political views, gender, and so on, caregiving, like sickness and death, is a great equalizer. When we offer care with compassion to address a need we observe, we rise above the differences that separate us.

You are part of something bigger than yourself. You, and the millions of other caregivers out there, are changing the world by your efforts. The merit of your effort ripples outward, benefiting others in unknown and mysterious ways. It is difficult to imagine where we would be as a species if it was not for caregiving. I don't think we would be here if it were not for caregiving, the highest expression of our humanity. And it can feel impossible at times. However, we humans are good at making the impossible possible. It is simply what we do.

How to Use This Book

This book is organized into four sections: Mindfulness, Compassion, Loss, and Intimacy. Each section begins with two quotes from notable teachers. Within each section are several short chapters covering topics relevant to the caregiving experience. While I recommend reading the book sequentially, from beginning to end, each chapter stands on its own and can be used for quick interventions to address a particular caregiving challenge you may be facing.

Each chapter includes an opening Gatha, or verse, to remind you of your potential for calm and resilience. You can think of the Gathas as practice tools to help you maintain an attitude that supports your best care, both for your loved one and for yourself. These passages can be viewed as prayers, poems, mantras, or short pep talks. You can carry a Gatha with you to inspire you and remind you in the midst of any challenge that there is a different way to approach your caregiving.

At the end of each chapter you will find a practice activity, a simple meditation or exercise you can work with to strengthen your mindfulness, support your caregiving, and enhance your sense of well-being. These activities should not require too much of your time. However, the more time you spend with them, the more impactful they will be. Consider keeping a journal to record your observations and thoughts about the practice activities or what you read.

Finally, a resource section at the end of the book lists organizations and websites that will provide additional support for your caregiving.

If you discover useful resources not included that you think would be beneficial to others, please let me know for inclusion in future editions. You can share the resources with me at roy.remer@zencaregiving.org.

May this book help you discover comfort and ease in your caregiving.

MINDFULNESS

The mindful path is the one that reveals itself as you walk down it. You cannot find the path until you step on to it.

— Kelly McGonigal

Every morning when we wake up, we have twenty-four brand-new hours to live. What a precious gift! We have the capacity to live in a way that these twenty-four hours will bring peace, joy, and happiness to ourselves and others.

— Thich Nhat Hanh

CHAPTER 1

Why Mindfulness

This moment this breath
Complete just as it is
This is where I can rest
Right here right now

This chapter makes a case for integrating mindfulness into your caregiving and into your life generally. Mindfulness and meditation are defined, and their relationship is presented. You will learn how to reclaim control of situations that cause stress and chaos.

Why should you trust that mindfulness can help in your caregiving? In recent years, studies looking at the benefits of mindfulness have increased significantly. According to the American Mindfulness Research Association, the number of journal articles on mindfulness increased from one in 1982 to 1,153 in 2020. (And since 2020 there has been a huge proliferation of studies on the effects of mindfulness.) This huge increase in the attention paid to the potential benefits of mindfulness practice on human well-being confirms what has been assumed for more than 2,500 years by practitioners of wisdom traditions teaching meditation and mindfulness. Applying scientific methods to understand the impact of mindfulness is a wonderful thing. Evidence is always good.

Recently, Zen Caregiving Project partnered with a team of

researchers from the Betty Irene Moore School of Nursing at the University of California at Davis to conduct a study looking at the benefits of our online Mindful Caregiving Education for family caregivers. While the caregiver course covers a variety of topics, we ground everything we do in mindfulness practice. The study found that the four-week online Mindful Family Caregiving course was associated with statistically significant decreases in symptoms of depression, anxiety, and caregiver burden and with increases in positive affect or well-being. There was also evidence of increased physical and emotional health in caregivers. And while it is still early days for research on mindfulness, most studies point to the potential benefits of mindfulness for mitigating the negative impacts of living in the modern world.

Trust plays a big role in deepening our ability to cultivate mindfulness. In my many years of practicing meditation and mindfulness, I have depended on conviction to keep me committed to my practice. This trust comes from what I have read and learned directly from meditation teachers from a variety of traditions. And with many years of experience behind me, I can say that meditation has changed my life. I would even say it has saved my life.

As a child and into my mid-twenties, I was a chronic worrier. When I was about six years old, I spent time in the hospital after missing many days of school due to chronic stomachaches. What my parents suspected was an ulcer was diagnosed as "nervous stomach." I was often in the grips of anxiety. Things improved in my teen years, but stomach issues have always plagued me. It was not until I began meditating in my twenties that I learned how to manage stress and interrupt thoughts that triggered strong emotions and their disruptive physical manifestations. Let's look more closely at what I have come to view as a transformative intervention.

Defining Meditation and Mindfulness

I use the term *meditation* alongside *mindfulness*. Although you may be somewhat familiar with these words, let's begin our journey by defining them. A definition of *mindfulness* that I find most useful is *a flexible state of mind in which you are paying attention to the present moment, on purpose and without judgment.* I think I first read this definition in the works of Jon Kabat-Zinn, a physician and longtime meditator who was one of the first teachers to apply mindfulness practice outside the context of the meditation hall. His work developing what he calls mindfulness-based stress reduction has helped spread the impact of mindfulness practice.

Paying attention to the present moment points you toward noticing or observing what is right here, right now. You can rest your present-moment awareness on physical sensations, emotions, thoughts, or the immediate environment around you. This type of awareness is direct experience. That is to say, as soon as the mind becomes distracted by thoughts of past or future, resistance or speculation, you are no longer directly experiencing the present moment. It's good to remember that distraction is normal, so paying attention "on purpose" means developing the ability to notice when you become distracted. Once you notice distraction, you can direct your attention back to your present-moment experience, without judgment. Responding with kindness, return to what is right here, right now.

Over the years, observing my own patterns of mind, I have realized how distant most of us are from our own lives. Life is passing by, and we are missing it. Minutes, hours, and days go by, and we are checked out, thinking about what happened yesterday or anticipating what may happen tomorrow. Especially in the context of caregiving, rumination and worry are huge contributors to stress. I often catch myself spinning out into some worst-case scenario of what could happen with the person I am caring for. Through meditation, I have learned to keep coming back to what is right here, right now when I notice my distraction.

Most definitions of *meditation* describe it as a form of contemplation, which I find somewhat misleading. Meditation is contemplation to the extent that the object of our contemplation is the present moment. We are observing what is happening here and now. When you truly contemplate your present-moment experience, free of distracting thoughts of the past or future, you break through to a state of oneness with present-moment phenomena. You could say that, in a moment of total presence, you become the sights, sounds, and smells around you. The thinking mind separates you from your environment. Yet in present-moment awareness, there is no separation.

Meditation is a practice that deepens mindfulness. When meditating, you are taking time out of your usual activities to cultivate the ability to keep coming back. Whereas mindfulness can be applied in any situation, meditation is the circumstance you create to consciously practice staying present. So you could say that meditation is an activity, while mindfulness is a state of mind. It is a bit like studying a foreign language: Meditation is similar to studying, and mindfulness is like using what you've learned to speak the language.

Although I remain committed to a daily meditation practice and encourage others to do the same, I have come to believe that we can nurture mindfulness without making time for formal meditation. If you choose to purchase a meditation cushion and a bell, and to designate a special place in your home for use in daily meditation, wonderful. It will be a good thing with many benefits. However, each of us is presented with many opportunities throughout our days to practice mindfulness.

Any activity you engage in is an opportunity to cultivate present-moment awareness. For instance, when you are doing some household chore, practice giving your full attention to the task. Notice when your mind gets distracted, and simply bring your attention back to the chore. Whatever the task at hand, you can choose to direct your full attention to it. How often do you engage in some activity while your mind is far away planning for some completely unrelated activity? This is completely normal, and yet it denies you of the benefits of resting your mind on what is right in front of you.

Reclaiming Control

When you take on a mindfulness practice, you will notice that the more you practice, the greater the benefits you will enjoy. And as stated, although meditation is the best way to practice mindfulness, it is not the only way. Use what you already do to practice mindfulness, and see if it changes the way you feel and cope with stressful situations.

Caregiving can be extremely demanding. It is common to feel overwhelmed by the number of things that need to get done. Even though the long list of things requiring your attention may not be optional, the stress of worrying about not accomplishing everything is. A distracted mind filled with worry is exhausting, yet a focused mind is the antidote to this exhaustion. You can choose to let go of the distracting thoughts causing anxiety, anger, and frustration. For instance, you can rest your attention on each motion involved with folding clothing, even though dinner still needs to be prepared and doctor's appointments need to be made. While you may not always feel you have control over your circumstances, you do have control over your mind state. You can use mindfulness to reclaim control of your state of mind and reclaim the ease that comes with it.

In the following chapters of part 1, you will learn ways to integrate mindfulness into your daily caregiving activities. First let's look at a basic practice to get you started with practicing mindfulness.

[Practice]

Numerous studies have shown that taking three deep intentional breaths activates the parasympathetic nervous system that calms the mind and body. Even in a busy day filled with the demands of caregiving, work, and home life, it should be easy to find a moment to stop and follow three deep breaths.

- Wherever you are, whatever you are doing, simply pause and close your eyes. Let your attention shift to the subtle sensations of breathing in and breathing out.
- Breathe in through your nostrils, deeply into your belly, and out through your mouth.
- If you want to extend this meditation for three more breaths,

try observing without attempting to alter the rhythm of your breathing
- See if you can do this at intervals throughout the day.

This simple, quick practice is a great way to reset when you notice you are overly distracted or experiencing agitation. Start from exactly where you are, right here, right now. Let each moment and each breath be an opportunity to begin again.

CHAPTER 2

This Perfect Moment

No past no future
Right here right now
Resting in the truth
Of this present moment

At the center of everything there is a stillness, a place of calm that is always within reach. No matter what is going on within or around you, that stillness waits to be found. This chapter explains how to find peace in each moment, regardless of your circumstances.

Caregiving can be extremely chaotic and stressful. As a caregiver, you are focused on the needs of others. It may feel impossible to accomplish all that is asked of you and still show up fully for every interaction or situation. Despite the demands, you can find a place of stillness and rest your mind there. How do you find that stillness? By coming back to the present moment.

Let's revisit the definition of mindfulness covered in the last chapter. *Mindfulness is a flexible state of mind in which you are paying attention to the present moment on purpose, without judgment.* When you pay attention to whatever is happening right here, right now, you strengthen your ability to return to a mind state of present-moment awareness, no matter what you are doing or what is unfolding around you. Coming back from distracting thoughts is possible at any moment, in any situation. If mindfulness was only achievable in the quiet moments when you get to take a break, it would not really be all that useful. The more you practice dropping into present-moment awareness, the easier it becomes to access it when life becomes chaotic.

Coping with Stress

Moments of chaos or heightened stress are not just unpleasant; they can be unhealthy when they reach such a high level that you no longer believe you have the resources to effectively cope. Everyone experiences stress. Some stress is actually healthy, since it stimulates your mind and motivates you. Although the perception of stress differs from one person to the next, health professionals agree that constant heightened stress is extremely unhealthy.

The good news is that mindfulness is a beneficial resource you can add to your defenses against unhealthy levels of stress. In addition to external caregiving resources like getting more assistance, additional training, or newer equipment or internal resources like more knowledge or physical fitness, maintaining present-moment awareness will strengthen your resilience and thus your sense of well-being.

You've probably heard a lot recently about resilience, since it has become a buzzword in healthcare. We can define *resilience* as our ability to bounce back from life's challenges, including but not limited to adversity, vulnerability, and loss and grief. Recognizing the burden all caregivers carry, health systems have made progress in providing resources that support increased resiliency.

We all know what it feels like to be our best selves. I encourage you to take a moment to think about what it feels like when you are at your best. When you feel at the "top of your game," what is going on in your mind? What is going on in your body? Maybe close your eyes and let yourself follow two to three inhales and exhales. Then take a moment or two to consider the experience of feeling your best. You probably recalled moments of heightened engagement, availability, joy, and ease. This is the mind state you return to when you bounce back from challenges and experience resilience. And you can support this mind state by staying engaged in present-moment awareness.

A study conducted in India in 2015 with college students looked at the relationship between mindfulness, resilience, and a sense of well-being and found that resilience plays an important role in the relationship between mindfulness and well-being. The greater one's ability to access mindful awareness, the easier it is to bounce back from challenging situations. And the easier it is for someone to bounce back from challenging situations, the greater their sense of happiness and well-being.

Sticky Mind

In chapter 4 we will look more closely at using mindfulness to deal with challenging circumstances. For now, let's consider a mind state that contributes to stress. I call this state "sticky mind," or having a particular thought that gets stuck and won't let go. Although a sticky mind often occurs when your thoughts are focused on the past, it can also take place when you are apprehensive about the future. In this state, your thoughts replay again and again. Sticky mind has a way of persisting, and you may not even realize it.

Rumination, a form of sticky mind, is a common issue for many people. It is natural to think about what we said, what we could have said, or what we did not say. Or to think about what others did or did not say. Or to think about something that happened in the past. This is especially true when something was said or when something happened that we were not happy about.

The same is true with apprehension. Thinking about the future to prepare for something unpleasant or to be ready for something unknown is very common. Apprehension is especially prevalent when caring for someone living with a serious illness. You likely worry about how things will unfold. *What will happen? How bad will it be? Will I be able to deal with it?*

I am sure you have experienced sticky mind many times yourself.

I was especially moved by a story of a spouse caregiver that illustrates well the suffering that sticky mind can cause. Angela recently attended one of our classes on mindful caregiving and shared a common issue faced by people caring for someone living with dementia. She spoke about her experience of moving her husband into a memory care facility when she could no longer safely care for him at home. Angela shared that she was finding it impossible to let go of regret. Although she was still healthy herself, she was exhausted and could not protect her husband from hurting himself in their home. Nonetheless, she continued to turn over in her mind the decision to relocate her husband and possible scenarios that could have enabled him to stay home. She considered bringing him home since he was very unhappy living in an unfamiliar environment, even though she knew that by all measures he was now safer, with twenty-four-hour care. Her distress was obvious as she tried her best to hold back tears while telling her story.

When I asked her what she does with these thoughts when they arise, Angela explained that sometimes she does not even realize she is having them. When she catches herself, she tries to find a distraction or thinks about visiting or calling her husband. I explained that something she could do, though it wouldn't make the pain of the difficult circumstances go away, is to return to what is true in the moment. As a class, we tried it together. We paused to follow a few breaths and acknowledge the experience of being together right here, right now.

This is the gift of the present moment when you catch yourself ruminating or having apprehensive thoughts. You just come back to what is right here, right now. Again and again. In this way, you will be disrupting thoughts that serve no positive purpose. You have the power to choose where you direct your attention, to thoughts that create more stress or to an awareness of what is actually happening in the moment. This is how you learn to bounce back. Though it is a simple process, it is not always easy to maintain. It takes vigilance and effort. This is why we refer to working with mindfulness as a practice.

Benefits of Mindfulness

As you practice coming back to the present moment, you will begin to enjoy three primary benefits of mindfulness: *calm mind*, *increased concentration*, and *heightened awareness*. Let's look at each of these in turn in the context of caregiving.

Calm Mind

As you practice, your mind will become calmer and steadier since you will begin to spend less time caught in the type of thoughts that cause agitation. This more grounded state of being will enable you to respond skillfully to what people say and to difficult situations so that the tension of the situation can be minimized. A calm mind supports clearer thinking. Also, when you are calm, you have a calming effect on those around you. This calming influence on the person you care for can be especially beneficial. In chapter 6, we will look at how this works.

Increased Concentration

With mindfulness, or paying attention on purpose, you notice when your attention is pulled away by distracting thoughts. It is impossible to avoid distracting thoughts, since the brain is constantly generating them. Please don't think you are failing if you keep noticing that you are distracted by random thoughts. The very fact that you are noticing means you are becoming more mindful. And, as you become more mindful, you will catch yourself more quickly when you become distracted, making it easier to concentrate on what you are doing. By improving your ability to concentrate, you reduce the likelihood of human error. This is extremely important when it comes to caregiving tasks like providing hands-on assistance with physical needs, managing medications, and recording important medical instructions. A focused mind is a less exhausted mind. You will find you are able to sustain more energy when you can maintain your attention on what you are doing or the person you are talking to.

Heightened Awareness

Although reviewing past mistakes to learn from them, or thinking about a future event so as to be adequately prepared, can be helpful, most of the time the thoughts we have about the past or future are not at all beneficial. The increased awareness that comes from cultivating mindfulness includes noticing more quickly when you are engaged in thinking that serves no positive purpose. The earlier you catch and disrupt negative thoughts, the easier it will become to shift your focus and engage in positive thinking or at least abide in a mind state that does not cause harm. Also, increased awareness helps maintain healthy self-care since you will be more attuned to what is happening in your body, and you will notice potential health issues before they become serious.

Increased present-moment awareness entails not only self-awareness but also awareness of the environment around you. Heightened awareness makes it easier to notice things in the environment that may have a negative effect on the person you are caring for. If you care for someone who is no longer able to express themselves, this kind of awareness can be very useful in ensuring their optimal comfort. Many years ago, when I was working in a healthcare facility, I heard a low-level noise in the hallway. When I asked a resident if they could hear it too, they shared that the sound bothered them. We addressed the issue easily, making the resident feel much more comfortable.

When the person you care for is nonverbal, your increased awareness will support your sensitivity to their nonverbal communication, such as facial expressions, body language, and the sounds they make. We will address this type of sensitivity more fully in chapter 27 when we look at healing touch.

Mindfulness Enhances Your Care

Mindfulness benefits not only you but also the kind of care you provide. This is one of the things I have appreciated most about practicing Zen and mindfulness over the years, the way my practice is not limited to my own experience but has enhanced my relationships with others.

When you are able to drop into present-moment awareness when offering care, you establish the conditions that support deep human connection. Others sense when you are lost in distraction, and they also notice when you are fully present. Apart from relief from physical pain, I have come to believe that what humans long for most when living with illness is the experience of deep connection. We are relational beings, and while deep human connection alone may not be curative, it allows someone living with an illness to feel a sense of wholeness, a sense of being part of something bigger than themselves. Deep connection supports emotional healing.

Toward the end of my mother's life, during one visit I decided to try something new in how I spent time with her. I often felt that my mother could see me only as the young boy who still lived with her and my father. Sometimes this was really nice, and at other times I felt unseen by her. And, if I am honest, I could only really see her as my mother. That is to say, I didn't really think about her as a person who had a life and an identity apart from being a mother to me and my siblings. On this particular day, I set an intention to see my mother differently, as another human being experiencing the challenges of living with serious illness and to not let our unique relationship influence the way I engaged with her. I wanted to maintain present-moment awareness, despite whatever she said or did that was either rooted in our past relationship or was challenging for me to accept.

The visit ended up being one of the best experiences I remember having with my mother toward the end of her life. Without my explaining to her what I was doing, she seemed to be meeting me in present moment. I think she felt really witnessed and supported by how I was showing up. We were two human beings paying close attention and meeting each other without regret or expectation.

Reflecting on the visit so many years after her death, I feel a profound sense of gratitude for my mindfulness practice that allowed me to connect so deeply with my mother before she died. This is a reminder of how each unfolding moment can be a gift, if we are fully available for what it holds. I hope you will have similar experiences of present-moment connection with the person you care for.

[Practice]

Set an alarm for once or twice a day. The amount of time you set is not important. Regardless of where you are or what you are doing when your alarm goes off, return to present-moment awareness. Give your attention fully to whatever you are doing. See how long you can maintain your mindful awareness without getting pulled away by distracting thoughts.

Keep practicing in this way. Try setting the alarm for more times during the day. You will begin to see that it gets easier to return to and maintain present-moment awareness. Notice if this has any impact on the way you experience stress. Before you know it, you won't need to set an alarm as a reminder. Returning to what is right here, right now, will become quite natural.

CHAPTER 3

The Refuge of Sensing Mind

This breath
This sensation
An opportunity to begin again
Starting from exactly where I am

Most of us live our lives a short distance from our body, to borrow a phrase from the writer James Joyce. We have been blessed with remarkable brains, which can process an astounding amount of information at once. Yet our ability to process so much information actually contributes to much of our stress and exhaustion. In this chapter we look at how you can use the body to rest your busy mind and disrupt any thoughts that cause stress.

In chapter 2, we looked at coming back to the present moment when we experience sticky mind, a mind state in which we can't let go of certain thoughts. If you are anything like me, you probably also experience a mind state often referred to as "monkey mind," or thinking about many things at once. In this mind state your thoughts quickly bounce from one topic to another. It is no surprise that when a lot is expected of you, you are more likely to experience this monkey mind. Although we're all capable of experiencing extended periods of this kind of overloaded thinking, monkey mind has a negative impact on your ability to focus and can be exhausting. When you are stuck in any kind of negative thinking, living life a short distance from your body, you miss the opportunity to focus on your body as a way to rest your busy mind.

Thinking Mind Versus Sensing Mind

You can learn to differentiate between brain activity that analyzes information and brain activity that simply perceives what is happening. When you process information, you could say you are activating the *thinking mind*, and when you perceive phenomena, you are activating the *sensing mind*. We all have the ability to know when we are sensing something without evaluating it.

Here is an example that illustrates the difference between thinking mind and sensing mind. Let's say you take a break from what you are doing to step outdoors for a moment. You close your eyes and just listen to the sounds around you. You hear some familiar sounds, but then you hear something unfamiliar. You may let yourself simply experience the unfamiliar sound, or you may get curious and begin trying to figure it out, where it is coming from, when it will end, why you've never heard it before. The direct experience of hearing a sound is sensing mind, while analyzing the sound is thinking mind. The inquiry about the sound takes you out of the present moment.

You can learn to shift between thinking mind and sensing mind to minimize stress. The thinking mind is essential in understanding the world we live in. It supports learning from past experiences, integrating new information, and planning for the future. The sensing mind is equally important. It allows you to observe what is happening in this very moment in your body and in the environment around you. It allows you to rest the busy mind. Although becoming familiar with noticing the difference between these two states of mind can be challenging, it is useful to learn how to shift from thinking mind to sensing mind when you need to enhance a sense of ease and well-being.

Metacognition

Through mindfulness practice, you cultivate the ability to step into the role of observer of your own mind state. Instead of being swept away in thoughts, you begin to notice what you are thinking. This noticing is a form of mindful awareness and is known as metacognition. Perhaps you recall a time when you had a disagreement with someone. The encounter ended, yet you continued to rehash the situation. The thought is sticking and just won't let go. It is safe to say the recurring thought distracts you from fully focusing on anything else. The moment you realize you are stuck in these thoughts, you become aware of your own mind state. This is stepping back and observing yourself. This is a moment of activating the sensing mind, when you can reset your thinking and your attention.

When you activate the sensing mind, you are in present-moment awareness. You can step back to notice not only your thoughts but also your emotions (which we will address in a later chapter) and your physical sensations. When you observe physical sensations, you are directly experiencing phenomena as they unfold; you are in the present moment. The sensations you are experiencing right now have nothing to do with the past or the future. It is only when you build a story about what you observe that you move back into the thinking mind and into either the past or the future.

The practice activity in chapter 1 guided you to focus on your breath and is an excellent way to drop into the sensing mind. Your breath is always with you wherever you go. It is always there for you when you need help returning to the present moment. The breath, and your physical sensations, are doorways into mindful awareness.

Cycle of Distraction

As you work with mindfulness, you will likely begin to notice a cycle. Let's say you pause to follow your breath for a moment or two. You start off with curiosity about the simple act of breathing in and breathing out. Then, after a few breaths, you notice you've become distracted by a thought. You let go of the thought and return to noticing your breath. This cycle repeats and is a natural part of learning mindfulness.

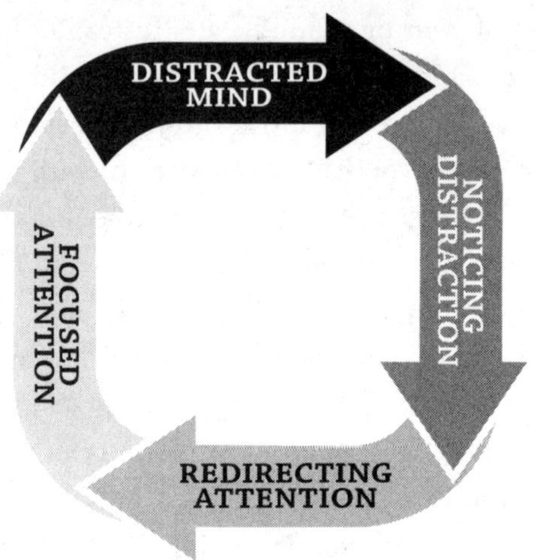

The key to resting in the sensing mind is to notice as soon as you begin thinking about what you are sensing. When you begin to create a story about what you are sensing, you are slipping back into the thinking mind. As soon as you become aware of your thinking, see if you can let go of the thought and return to pure observation. Staying with observation without thinking about what you observe may not be easy at first, but it will get easier as you practice.

Though you may at first feel frustrated when you notice you are distracted (again), it is actually a really good thing. It is the experience of noticing that begins to build new neural connections in the brain, giving you the tools necessary to manage stress effectively and provide better care.

Take a moment to imagine a caregiving situation that causes you stress or anxiety. Notice what thoughts or strong emotions arise for you. Now, after thinking about the scenario for a moment or two, let go of thoughts about the scenario and redirect your attention fully to your breath. Rest here, following the breath. As soon as you notice yourself beginning to form thoughts about inhaling and exhaling, try to let go of these thoughts, and fully return to observing the sensations associated with the act of breathing. After a few moments of focusing on the breath, notice what your feet feel like in contact with your socks or with the floor. Again, if you notice distracting thoughts, let them go and return to sensations. Finally, if you are sitting down, notice the parts of your legs in contact with the chair beneath you.

When turning your attention to the sensations in the body, you will likely become more aware of physical discomforts. If you observe a discomfort in your lower back, for instance, you may begin to wonder what is causing it. You may begin to worry about how bad it could get. Or you may ask yourself, *Did I do something to cause this discomfort? Do I need to take some aspirin? Could it be my kidneys? Will I be able to get an appointment with my doctor?* Before you know it, you are solidly back in the thinking mind. This is all very natural, but it is also optional.

Choosing Where to Direct Your Attention

Of course, addressing a perceived problem in the body is extremely important. However, you can choose when to problem-solve and when to rest in present-moment awareness of what is happening in the body. Rather than problem-solving the discomfort, or trying to escape it, you might instead get really curious about the sensations. You may be able to accept the discomfort for only a moment or two, but that is a great start. You could also try shifting your observation from the area of discomfort to a spot that is not uncomfortable.

By now you might be asking yourself why this is useful. What does all this have to do with caregiving? Caregiver stress and anxiety are often caused by thinking about issues beyond your control. When you are caring for someone, it is very natural to think about the progression of their illness or even what may have caused the illness. You may feel a need to know what happens next. Projecting yourself into the future has its place, but dwelling too much on unknowns can cause suffering. In addition, such thinking does not do much good for the person you are caring for, since thinking about the future or the past takes you away from that person. When your thoughts are elsewhere, those around you can tell; they feel your absence.

When you come back to what is true in the moment, you disrupt the thoughts that cause stress and anxiety. Coming back again and again to the immediacy of physical sensations, you reinforce your calm and steady mind. You give your thinking mind a rest and strengthen connection to the person you are caring for. Learning to use the sensing mind as a refuge from busy thoughts is moment-by-moment self-care. It is healthy for you — and for those you care for.

[Practice]

Let yourself pause during the day. Close your eyes, and observe the difference between the thinking mind and the sensing mind.

- Find a quiet spot to sit, and close your eyes.
- Observe the thoughts that arise for you as you stop for a moment.
- Now let your attention shift from observing thoughts to observing sensations. You might begin by noticing the sensations that are part of inhaling and exhaling.
- Then see what other sensations you can observe in your body. If you observe a sensation that you find unpleasant, see if you can stay with it for a few more breaths, or move to some other sensation.
- As soon as you begin to create a story or to think about the sensation you observe, see if you can let go of those thoughts and return to direct experience of the sensation itself: What does coolness feel like? Heat? Pressure? Soreness? Fatigue? Your skin in contact with your clothing?
- How curious can you be about the sensations in your body?
- Spend as much time as you can exploring the dynamic between your sensing mind and your thinking mind.

When you finish, think about what this direct experience of sensations was like. Did it feel different from focusing on your thoughts? Continue to practice shifting from thoughts, especially thoughts that are not useful, to sensations. You can always choose when to let go of your thoughts.

CHAPTER 4

Being with Challenging Circumstances

I am only human
Making the impossible possible
Is what we humans do

Caregiving is fraught with uncertainty. From one moment to the next, you may not know what will be expected of you. Illness, and the emotions it elicits, can be unpredictable. Though you may want to know, we rarely know what to expect when a loved one is suffering. In this chapter, we will look at how you can use mindfulness to cope with the uncertainty and discomfort of difficult situations.

Honesty about What Is Happening

Hopefully, you are beginning to see that mindfulness is about honesty and authenticity. In present-moment awareness, we observe what is actually happening. When I encounter something challenging, I begin by acknowledging that the situation is tough, messy, or uncomfortable. I remind myself that there is no room for pretending: This is what is here, so let's deal with it. In some situations I may even say out loud to the person I am with, who may be contributing to the challenging situation, "This is really uncomfortable."

The most important thing is to be honest with yourself and proceed from there. Of course, challenging situations take many different forms. While you can readily address some situations with a clear solution, you may best address others by simply staying mindful with an open heart. You can be sure things will change because everything changes with the passage of time, so responding from the heart and simply being with the situation is a really effective approach.

Openhearted presence is often underrated as a strategy for dealing with challenging circumstances. You have probably heard the saying "Don't just sit there, do something!" I think there are plenty of situations where the Zen spin on this is the better approach: "Don't just do something, sit there!" Sometimes doing nothing is exactly what is called for. When I am faced with a challenge, I remind myself of something I heard Charlie Garfield, the founder of Maitri Hospice in San Francisco, say: "Forget about improving things, just don't make it worse." Although we may want to improve a situation, it may in fact be beyond our control, and we need to meet the situation as it is.

Fixing Is Overrated

Rather than immediately getting busy with action, it can be useful to pause long enough to discern whether action would be helpful or whether openhearted presence alone is what is called for. Being too focused on fixing a problem can actually create distance between you and the person you believe needs to hear a solution. Perhaps you have had the experience of sharing a problem with a friend who immediately moves into ways of addressing the problem. This feels really different from sharing with a friend who will listen deeply and wait until they are asked for ideas.

Many of us identify with being helpful, so we quickly move into fix-it mode when we encounter something challenging. Helping others has a way of making us feel good about who we are. Yet moving too quickly into helping can be disempowering for the person we think needs help. There is nothing wrong with assisting when it is requested or when we are certain the person we care for has no way of managing the situation on their own. When we encounter a loved one struggling with discomfort or big emotions, we might ask, "Would you like some help with this, or would you prefer I just be with you?" The main point here is that instead of moving immediately into helping, consider the option of simply being a companion to a loved one with a problem.

Marilyn is a woman I visit regularly as a volunteer. She suffers from a rare chronic illness that causes intense pain throughout her body. When Marilyn shares how overwhelmed she feels by all the logistical issues related to her many medical needs, I notice my mind moving into problem-solving. However, when I step back, I become convinced that the best way to support her is by offering openhearted attention and not solutions. I try to let go of fixing her problems and instead settle into deep listening. When I get caught up in figuring out ways to address her challenges, I am no longer really with her. I may still be sitting beside her, but my mind is far away. Every now and then I ask if she wants some ideas on how to cope with the overwhelm, but I know that is not actually why I am there. If she asks me what I think she should do, then I let my mind move into problem-solving.

Calming Your Own Agitation

Encountering a difficult situation can cause a lot of agitation. Your heart rate may increase, you may begin to feel warm or sweaty, you may feel a surge of energy in your limbs, or perhaps you even feel like screaming out loud. Such physical sensations may make it difficult to discern what is most needed. So, as with the techniques presented in the last chapter, in these moments try to direct your attention to these sensations. Getting really curious about where in your body you are experiencing emotions and resting attention there has a way of quieting the physical sensations.

When I am struggling, I have found it is also useful to say to myself, "Okay, I've got this. I can handle this situation." This expression of self-soothing helps build the confidence to stay present even amid a difficult situation. Self-compassion, which we will look at in chapter 12, is another extremely supportive form of self-soothing.

When encountering extreme suffering in the person or people you care for, or any kind of difficult situation, you may feel a desire to run away. You may even feel panic coming on. In such moments you might try coaching yourself to stay for one more breath. And then another. And another...This focus on the breath will help you calm down and stay put. Staying for one more breath may seem like a small thing, yet it will take down the intensity of the experience almost instantly.

Though you never know when or where it will happen, you can be certain that sooner or later you will find yourself feeling very uncomfortable or unprepared. It is easier to accept that this is a normal part of life and of caregiving when you know there are tools you can use in such situations. And shifting into mindful awareness is one of the best tools to use when you feel like things are spinning out of control.

I will never forget when I was asked to sit with a woman experiencing extreme restlessness and confusion, otherwise known as terminal agitation. The nursing assistants had created a padded enclosure around her to keep her safe because she would flail about and attempt to climb out of bed. I was asked to stay by her bedside and keep her from injuring herself. I was initially overwhelmed by what I was seeing and filled with doubt that I could do anything to help. After that initial resistance and sense of helplessness, I found my way into some deep breathing. Speaking to her softly and redirecting her active limbs, I did my best to keep part of my attention on my own body. I spent a few hours with the woman until she finally exhausted herself and fell into a fitful sleep. Mindfulness may not prevent a difficult situation, but it will help maintain stability and confidence until the situation, like everything else, transforms into something else.

[Practice]

You can use past difficult situations to help you prepare for the next time things start to feel out of control. You can also practice imagining a scenario that you may encounter in the future.

- Take a moment to focus on your breath.
- Once you have grounded yourself in present-moment awareness, try recalling a recent situation you found difficult or thinking of something you anticipate encountering in the future. It could be the person you are caring for expressing a big emotion or a disagreement with a loved one, or perhaps you had to do something you felt unprepared for. Any challenging situation will do.
- Imagine yourself attuning to the breath while in the midst of the situation.
- Then offer yourself some self-coaching or soothing words of encouragement.
- If you are recalling a situation where there was nothing you could do to change the outcome, imagine telling yourself that you accept that nothing can be done to fix the situation.
- Return to maintaining attention on the breath for a moment or two.

Following the practice, take a few moments to reflect on how things felt different or the same. You might write down a note or two on how it felt to apply some mindful awareness and self-soothing in the midst of the situation you recalled.

CHAPTER 5

Working Skillfully with Big Emotions

In each moment
I choose how to meet whatever arises
My experience and my choice

This chapter shows you how to stay grounded and present when you have a big emotional reaction. We will discuss the importance of emotions and how they function. And you will discover how to build your capacity for allowing emotions to show up without disrupting your sense of connection or the care you provide.

When dropping into present-moment awareness, you can direct your attention toward internal or external stimulus, such as your thoughts, your physical sensations, your emotions, or the immediate environment around you. Let's look at building self-awareness of emotions and how to manage the experience of activated emotions. If you are not used to working with your emotions, you may feel like they are in control. Emotions can be powerful, difficult, even painful. They shape our experience. However, by cultivating the ability to step back and notice your moment-by-moment experience, you learn that you can choose how to respond to heightened emotions when they arise. By applying mindful awareness to emotions arising in the body and mind, you take away their potentially disruptive power.

Defining *Emotion*

While there seems to be little scientific consensus on what an emotion is, I find it useful to think of emotions as part thought and part physical sensation. The American Psychological Association defines emotions as "conscious mental reactions (such as anger or fear) subjectively experienced as strong feelings usually directed toward a specific object and typically accompanied by physiological and behavioral changes in the body." However we define emotions, we can observe the direct interplay between thoughts and physical sensations.

It is normal to feel swept away by your emotions. Let's say you regret your behavior after having a big reaction to something someone said or did. On reflection you realized you let yourself be controlled by your emotions. Maybe in the moment you felt helpless against them. This is very natural, and everyone experiences this from time to time. When we are not aware of the impact emotions have on our actions, it is easy to lose control of our behavior.

There is nothing wrong with emotions, whether they are strong or subtle, positive or negative. Emotions allow us to feel moved by the world around us, and they help us stay safe. In fact, they have played an essential role in our evolution, helping humans survive and develop. When you practice mindfulness, you should not be concerned that you will lose the richness of emotional experience. Mindfulness allows you to fully experience an emotion without reacting to it unskillfully. With practice, you will become more adept at choosing how to respond to emotions while experiencing them fully.

An emotional reaction to what you perceive through your senses can be instantaneous. There is really no way to prevent, say, a startle reaction when you suddenly sense something that may cause you harm. While walking down a creek bed in a desert canyon a few years ago, I almost stepped on a rattlesnake. Before I understood what the sound of the rattle represented, I jumped back. I didn't think to jump, I just jumped. The signal my ears detected was processed instantly in one part of my brain, which caused an automatic reaction. Another part of my brain processed the information it received and helped me understand it was a snake. I was then able to slowly back away while speaking softly. The more primal part of my brain that processes messages in a fraction of a second made me act before I actually understood what was happening. There was no way to control this type of fear reaction. And that was a good thing, since it can save you from being bitten by a poisonous snake!

Rather than looking at the emotions that arise when your physical safety is threatened, I will focus here on how to respond to less immediate threats like caregiving challenges that impact your peace of mind or threaten your ego. It is common for people experiencing pain to react strongly when touched or moved. Certain types of dementia can cause angry outbursts. Finding oneself on the receiving end of anger can cause unintentional reactions. When it comes to challenges like unpleasant words or behavior directed at you, or situations that cause feelings of concern or sadness, you can learn new and healthy ways of responding.

Locating Emotions in the Body

Since we know that emotions are accompanied by a physiological change in the body, it is helpful to look at how different emotions show up in different parts of the body. See if your experience of each of these emotions aligns with any of their corresponding physical expressions:

- **Anger:** increased blood flow to the arms and hands. You might feel like you want to hit something or someone.
- **Fear:** increased energy in the main muscle groups of the body like the legs. You might feel like you want to run.
- **Surprise:** your eyebrows raising as if you are trying to take more into your field of vision
- **Anxiety:** a cramping or a loose feeling in the gut
- **Sadness:** sensations in the chest and shoulders that can feel like contractions. Grief can cause sensations of physical collapse.

- **Shame or embarrassment:** blushing cheeks or increased body heat and perspiration
- **Disgust:** contractions of facial muscles
- **Joy or happiness:** increased energy and mental activity

It is helpful to get really curious about how your own body expresses emotions. Learning to identify where emotions show up in your body will make it easier to direct attention there in the midst of an emotional reaction.

Lifecycle of an Emotion

Although the physical manifestations of certain emotions may be unpleasant, they can actually be used to shorten the duration of the emotion itself. A typical emotion does not last very long. In fact, an emotion lasts only a moment or two in the body and brain. If you are surprised by this, you are not alone. Emotions often feel like they linger for a long time. This is because the thoughts or memories that initially triggered the emotional response are repeated over and over, thereby making it difficult for the cycle to wind down.

When you are aware of your thoughts, you can catch yourself in a cycle that retriggers emotions. Once you catch yourself, then what? Upon noticing you are engaging in thinking that generates a particular emotion, direct your attention to the physical manifestation of the emotion. Get really curious about where the emotion is being expressed in the body, and what it feels like. As soon as you begin to layer thoughts on top of the physical sensations, try to let go of the thoughts and return to the direct experience of the sensations. You already practiced this in chapter 3. By maintaining your focus on the physical sensation associated with the emotion, you let the emotion play itself out, but you don't feed the emotion with additional thoughts. You are simply stepping back and observing, and this disrupts the thought-emotion cycle.

I am someone who is prone to anxiety. This has been true ever since I can remember. Recently, I have had moments of anxiety triggered by my inability to get in touch with my elderly father, who lives by himself. When he doesn't answer his phone, my mind immediately goes to what could be wrong. Worst-case scenarios flash through my mind. I immediately feel a sinking feeling in my gut. It is a familiar rumbling that at once feels tight and loose.

In these moments, I try to stop and just experience the physical sensations. If I give all my attention to the sensations associated with the anxiety, I am actually interrupting the thoughts that have caused the emotion in the first place. I am not denying the emotion, and I am not swept up in it. I am simply experiencing it without feeding it with continued unconscious or unaware thinking. I am using my body in this intervention, or returning to the sensing mind as a refuge. And I can more easily come up with a plan in case I do not hear back from him within a reasonable amount of time.

You Are More Than Your Emotions

I have found it helpful to acknowledge to myself that although I am feeling anxiety, I do not need to identify too closely with that emotion. Instead of saying to myself, "I am anxious" I might say, "Anxiety is here." Or, "This is an experience of anxiety." Or, "This is what anxiety feels like." This is another way to step back and observe what I am experiencing and can be done with any emotion.

As a caregiver, you may feel like you don't have time for strong emotions, since there is just too much to do. Or you may think making space for your emotions is somehow selfish and means you are not concerned about the person you are caring for. Perhaps you resist allowing your emotions to surface if you are holding a lot of fear, sadness, or anticipatory grief. Your resistance may come from believing that you must be "strong" and somehow model stoicism for the person you care for.

Another common concern is that if you open to strong feelings, they will be bottomless, and you will feel angry or heartbroken forever.

In reality, if you let an emotion express itself, it will dissipate more quickly. By moving toward the physical sensations associated with an emotion through honest observation, you build your capacity to be with any emotion when it arises. This will provide you with more stability and a clearer mind for caregiving.

An Emotion Is What It Is

I hope you are beginning to see that it is healthiest to let yourself fully investigate emotions as they arise. Being mindful means being honest with yourself, acknowledging what is really happening — right here, right now. And sometimes this means being honest with whomever you are interacting with. It can be helpful to take a breath or two and say to those around you, "In this moment, I am experiencing fear." Or, "I am feeling sad about what you are going through." This can open up an authentic conversation and permit others to acknowledge their emotions.

You honor your experience when you acknowledge an emotion that is arising. By sharing what is happening, you take some of the power away from the emotion. You are conveying to those around you that you can handle this. Emotional expression, or sharing that you are experiencing a strong emotion, is different from emotional collapse. With collapse, the emotion has taken over and you are overwhelmed, temporarily unable to show up for others' needs. When you can acknowledge and express emotion, you can still function and address the immediate needs of others, without being "needy" yourself.

As you gain more confidence in dealing with your own emotions, you will be better able to support others when they are having a big emotional experience. It will become easier to detect the signs that someone is struggling. When someone is living with an advancing illness, a lot of emotions can arise. If you want to get better at supporting the person you care for, start with yourself.

Developing a Language for Emotions

Emotions are complex, and it can be difficult to talk about them with clarity. Most of us do not have an extensive vocabulary to describe our emotions. I often find I am at a loss to accurately describe my emotional experience. It requires that I slow down and pay careful attention.

When asked about an emotional experience, most people will share what they think about the emotional experience rather than describing the felt qualities of the emotion. The more you practice noticing emotions and where they show up in the body, the easier it will become to talk about your emotional experience.

It is not possible to experience caregiving or life in general without experiencing the ups and downs that emotions bring. Even if you could eliminate emotions, I am not sure you would want to. Emotions protect us, make us feel alive, and help us see the beauty and poignancy of the world around us. Even when confronting a difficult emotional experience, it is possible to regain your composure and calm your mind. If you have felt burdened by big emotions, I encourage you to change your relationship with them. All it takes is turning inward and paying attention.

[Practice]

Pause during your day and notice the emotions you are experiencing. You may choose to do this when something happens that causes a big emotional response or when you have a moment or two of downtime. During the pause, get really curious about the physical manifestations of the emotion.

- Where are emotions being expressed in your body?
- How would you describe the sensations associated with the emotions?
- Do the sensations stay the same or change over time?

- What exact emotion caused the physical sensations you notice?
- What thoughts inform the emotions you are observing?

Following this inquiry, consider writing in your journal about what you notice. Over time, as you pause to practice awareness of emotions, see if you notice any change in the way emotions impact the way you feel about yourself, your circumstances, or how you interact with others.

CHAPTER 6

Modeling Presence

Strong winds may stir chaos around me
The solid ground on which I stand
Keeps me steady
Steady for myself and others

The greatest gift you can offer the person you care for is your calm presence. Even when things are not going well or they become chaotic, your ability to stay grounded enhances your care in many ways. In this chapter, we will look at the impact of your mindfulness practice on those around you.

In his wonderful book *The Naked Now*, the modern-day Christian mystic Richard Rohr conveys a story from the Gospel of Luke about Jesus visiting his friends Mary, Martha, and Lazarus:

> Martha was everything good and right, but one thing she was not. She was not present — most likely, not present to herself, her own feelings of resentment, perhaps her own martyr complex, her need to be needed. This is the kind of goodness that does no good! If she was not present to herself, she could not be truly present to her guests in any healing way, and spiritually speaking, she could not even be present to God. Presence is presence to presence.

Unfortunately, this description of Martha could be applied to many caregivers. Many of us have not learned how to step back and observe or create intimacy with our own minds. Until we learn this, we remain unaware of our spinning minds, and healing ourselves and others remains out of reach.

As a caregiver, the greatest gift you can offer the person you are caring for is your calm presence. Your ability to stay grounded even when things are not going well or when things become chaotic enhances your care in many ways.

Sharing Calm

I have learned a great deal about applying mindful awareness to caregiving from the spiritual teacher Frank Ostaseski, founder of Zen Hospice Project and author of *The Five Invitations*. Frank is a wonderful teacher, and I had the pleasure of serving with him while learning to become a caregiver to people at the end of life. I will always be grateful for his generosity in modeling calm and compassionate caregiving. Frank would often say, "All it takes is one person in the room to shift the energy." If one person is calm and openhearted, they invite others to also regulate their emotions and express kindness. This is the essence of the Zen caregiving approach: calm and kindness establish a field of healing energy for both the caregiver and the person receiving care.

Let's consider here the experience of empathy and what it tells us about how the mind states and emotions we witness in others can be contagious. Empathy is a mind state that responds to the perceived suffering of others. It entails both an emotional experience and the motivation to alleviate any perceived suffering. When you experience empathy, you experience in your body or mind the pain or discomfort that you assume is taking place for the person you are observing. Recent brain-imaging studies show strong evidence that when subjects observe others experiencing physical pain or various emotional states, the areas of the brain associated with direct experience of the physical or emotional state are activated.

As the brain attunes to another's emotional and physical state, two primary networks of the brain are activated, a "mentalizing" network and a network of "mirror neurons." From infancy, these neural networks are working to track and read signs of the people around us. Think of an infant who is attuned to its parent's facial expressions and responding accordingly. With our highly evolved brain networks functioning behind the scenes, we have become very adept at tracking unspoken messages that are conveyed, often subtly, by other humans. This is how we have avoided or prepared for people who might do us harm, and how we have moved toward those who can help us when needed. What we perceive about others can have a distinct impact on our energy and emotions if we are not paying attention to our mind and body.

Take a moment to recall a situation when you witnessed someone experiencing a strong emotion like anxiety or sadness. Do you recall feeling like you could relate to what they were experiencing? Perhaps you felt as though you could also feel the perceived emotion. This emotional resonance is perfectly natural and helps us feel more connected to those around us; however, it is useful to maintain awareness of what is happening with our own thoughts and physical sensations when we begin to feel the emotions we observe in others.

Recently, I experienced emotional resonance with a close friend of mine on the final morning of a trip we took together. This friend, a longtime meditator, is typically very calm and at ease. In this particular interaction, he was rushing to get on the road for a long drive home. There was a lot for him to accomplish before departing. I, on the other hand, was not in a hurry and woke up very calm. I could see he was "upregulated," in other words, in a heightened energetic state. After some time in his presence, I realized that I was beginning to feel agitated as well. Once I noticed my own increasingly agitated state, I applied some of the practices we've looked at in previous chapters. I checked in with my breath. I attuned to the sensations in my body. I checked in with my emotions and thoughts. This allowed me to recalibrate and return to a calmer and more grounded state. It took awareness and some vigilance to get there, and to stay there.

On another recent occasion, I was with my father upon his return home from a few days in the hospital following a medical procedure. He needed to integrate some new prescriptions into his usual daily medications. Sitting with him at the kitchen table as he updated his two-week pill organizer, I noticed him becoming increasingly frustrated. My father and I have a long history of heightened emotional interactions. I noticed myself slowly beginning to meet him in a state of impatience and agitation. A storm was brewing. As soon as I stepped back to observe the scenario playing out, I told myself, "My job here as a caregiver is to stay calm and be available to assist him if he asks for assistance." I turned to my mindfulness practices to model for him a calm presence. I didn't need to say anything about what I was doing to stay calm. In fact, if I had told him or suggested that he try calming down, he probably would have become even more agitated. As I think back on the experience, I trust that the calm my father witnessed in me helped keep him steady enough to see the task through to its completion. Even if I am wrong, I am absolutely certain that I did not make his situation worse.

This second example shows that emotional resonance works in both directions. If you don't pay attention, you might suffer from the same emotional agitation you witness in others. And yet, if you are paying attention and you consciously apply mindful awareness to calm your mind and body, you can positively influence someone who is experiencing heightened agitation. Without even vocalizing a suggestion to relax, which can be very triggering for some people, you can simply model calm and ease if it is your authentic experience. Others will sense your steadiness. "All it takes is one person in the room to shift the energy." You can become that one person. You can support the sense of well-being of the person you are caring for by modeling presence.

Letting Go of Toxicity

The benefits of your mindfulness practice will also extend to relationships outside your caregiving. Friends, family, and colleagues will begin to notice something shifting in you. Whether or not you intend it, others will notice your calmer and steadier way of being. It is also true that as you become more attuned to others' energy, you may begin to notice that certain people in your life — even when well-intentioned — are extremely draining and have a chronic negative impact on your well-being. These types of people are known as toxic, and we all have them in our lives. As your emotional resilience increases, you may find yourself asking, "Why do I keep this person in my life?" Sadly, no matter how much you model presence, some people will remain toxic. For your own emotional health, you may need to decide to pull away from such relationships. Making this kind of decision, and following through with it, may be difficult, but in the long run, you will be healthier and happier.

Showing Vulnerability

As mentioned earlier, mindfulness practice is about being honest with yourself. Sometimes this means admitting that you are really struggling with a particular emotion. Although you are acquiring new emotional skills and building resilience, you will still face challenges. You are only human, after all. One element of modeling presence is allowing yourself to be fully witnessed by the person you are caring for, or by others around you, in your state of vulnerability. This kind of modeling does two things. First, it reminds the person you are caring for that being human means experiencing vulnerability. Their circumstances are different, but they are not alone in their suffering. And second, it allows the person you are caring for to express kindness and caring to you.

Just because someone is living with an illness does not mean they no longer need to express care and support to others, even their caregiver. Jane Verity, the founder of Dementia Care International, identified five core emotional needs of peoples living with a dementia-related illness; however, I think they are relevant to anyone, whether or not they are living with illness. These five core needs are: (1) to feel needed and useful, (2) to have the opportunity to care, (3) to love and be loved,

(4) to have self-esteem boosted, and (5) to have the power to choose. Being honest about how you are feeling may give the person you care for the opportunity to experience the first four emotional needs.

When I first came across the five core emotional needs, I thought of Raj. I met Raj years ago, shortly after training to become a hospice volunteer. On my first shift, I was unsure of myself and quite intimidated. Raj's room door was open, so I knocked gently on the door frame and waited for him to acknowledge my presence. Inviting me into his room, he asked me to sit in one of the chairs near his bed. The man I met was of slight build with thick jet-black hair and a beaming smile. He wore loose pajamas and glasses. As I stumbled through my attempts to make conversation, it must have become obvious to him that I was pretty nervous. Raj began asking me questions in a soft and supportive manner. Immediately, I sensed that he was focused on making me feel comfortable in his presence. The tables were turned, and he was taking care of me, when I thought I was supposed to be there to care for him. We talked for a while before I realized that he was becoming sleepy. I excused myself and left so he could rest.

Out in the hallway again, I was amazed and amused by what had just happened. Raj challenged my assumptions of what it means to provide care. After that visit, I vowed to be open to being cared for by the people I was there to serve. Why would I ever want to deny someone living with a serious illness the opportunity to express care? Letting others care for us when we are caregiving requires that we first honestly acknowledge that we may in fact need a bit of emotional support. Accepting emotional support from the person we care for is a different way to model presence but is equally beneficial.

Being honest with yourself when you are struggling also means paying attention when you are emotionally overwhelmed. When you are nearing or in a state of emotional collapse, it is probably best to turn to someone other than the person you are caring for to find appropriate support. Knowing when to call on support from the person you care for is about recognizing the limits of what they can handle, given their circumstances.

Not everyone has a dependable social support network. Your unique situation may make it difficult to turn to others for support. Modeling a willingness to ask for help is beneficial for those around you to witness. It is difficult for many people to ask for support when they are struggling, often because they see asking for help as a sign of weakness. In reality, when you ask for help, you are demonstrating courage. In addition, when you ask for help, you are giving others the permission they need to ask for support when they need it.

Generating Good Merit

Everyone benefits from the support of others, whether or not they are living with an illness. Each morning when I meditate, I finish with a *dedication of merit* that I recite out loud. This is to acknowledge that my time and efforts in meditation have an impact beyond my own direct experience. Dedicating the merit is a practice I learned when I began serving as a volunteer caregiver. It can be used to acknowledge any endeavor that benefits others. A dedication of merit can be very personal or universal.

When you model presence as a caregiver, you are offering something positive to the people around you. As we know by now, commitment to your practice of cultivating mindful awareness has clear benefits for you but also for those whom you interact with. The time you spend cultivating mindfulness and applying it to your caregiving has merit and comes with its own rewards, in the form of greater ease of being and an enhanced sense of well-being. When you pay attention to your own body, mind, and emotions, you become a safe and easeful presence for anyone you interact with. Modeling presence enhances wellness and healing for all you encounter.

[Practice]

Look for opportunities to model presence. When you interact with someone who is displaying a noticeable emotional or physical agitation, use what you have learned so far to stay calm and attentive to both your own and the other person's energy. If you notice yourself beginning to mirror someone else's upregulated energy, remember to keep part of your attention on your breath and your physical sensations. Let someone else's energy be like a meditation bell, reminding you to drop into present-moment awareness. See if you notice any shift in the other person's energy or in how they interact with you.

CHAPTER 7

Mindful Communication

Bringing calm and clarity
May our conversation close the distance between us
Each of us feeling seen and supported

Enhancing deep connection with the person you are caring for through conversation can be challenging when they are experiencing physical or emotional discomfort. In this chapter we look at how you can weave mindful awareness into your conversations.

Deepening Connection Through Conversation

A few years back, I visited with Irene, a friend who had recently received a cancer diagnosis. This was toward the end of the Covid pandemic, and she had put off seeing a doctor out of concern for exposure to the virus. Irene was told she had esophageal cancer that had spread to other areas of her body. By the time she shared with me what was going on, the cancer had already progressed significantly. Sitting with her on her back porch on a cool but sunny morning, I was struck by how thin Irene had become and what a strain it was for her to talk.

Our conversation was one of the most difficult I have ever had. Irene had been very isolated during Covid, and now she was fast reaching a point where she had to rely on the support of others to address her basic needs. She conveyed that she knew she was nearing the end of her life. Irene was adamant that she wanted to remain in her apartment until she died and was asking for my help in making sure that she would not be transferred to a hospital under any circumstances.

The next several weeks were a roller-coaster as I helped provide and organize care for Irene. It was not easy providing care in her home; however, we did our best to honor her wishes. Despite all that followed, it was that initial conversation when she shared the reality of her situation and her clear wishes for her dying experience that I will never forget.

In that conversation, my only job was to be a calm and openhearted presence. I had never known anyone more sensitive to others' energy than Irene. I had always felt she could read my innermost thoughts before even I was aware of them. In addition to my calm, I wanted to support her by giving her the opportunity to consider her situation from every angle. And I wanted Irene to feel my commitment to the conversation. In other words, I wanted her to know that for however long I had for our conversation, I was with her 100 percent.

As I look back on that morning, I recall a feeling of deep connection and clarity. There was sadness, and some fear, but mostly a great sense of love between two friends. That was an experience in which I felt a profound gratitude for my ability to access mindful awareness even during a painful conversation.

Overcoming Distractions

Communicating while maintaining mindful awareness is not easy. We live in a time when deep connection in conversation is rare. Most of us have been conditioned in recent years to only feel a sense of connection to others when we are communicating via an electronic device. And these devices we rely on to stay connected to the people we care about most bombard us constantly with distractions, which can be very damaging to our mental health. Each time our phone buzzes to inform us of some new bit of information, we experience stimulation in the reward center of the brain. We receive a hit of dopamine, a neurotransmitter that stimulates feelings of satisfaction or joy. The more we receive this hit of dopamine, the more we crave the sort of satisfaction that comes from these small but mighty devices we carry with us everywhere. Most of us are subtly attuned to our devices, waiting for the next message or notification to come in. This subtle anticipation of electronic distractions makes it more difficult to focus on tasks. Our devices can be especially disruptive when we are in a one-on-one in-person conversation.

Sociologist and psychologist Sherry Turkle, author of *Reclaiming Conversation*, makes the case that our electronic devices, and the digital world in general, threaten the health of our relationships. Taking back control over the flow of communication coming to us through our devices and reclaiming authentic conversation in this day and age may feel like an act of rebellion. Integrating mindful awareness into communications means reclaiming authentic conversation.

Authentic conversation is an experience of deep connection, with everyone involved in the conversation feeling truly seen and supported. At Zen Caregiving Project, we teach generous listening skills. With this kind of conversational engagement, we listen as though we are the last person who will ever hear this particular story. We listen with our mind, body, and heart. I remember one volunteer caregiver saying he tried to listen with his belly as well as his ears, conveying his level of commitment to the conversation. In this approach to conversation, you can't help but listen for what really matters. To support our volunteer caregivers to engage deeply in conversation, free from digital distractions, we insist that they not carry their phone with them when visiting patients.

Three Qualities of Mindful Communications

Years ago, thinking of ways to integrate mindfulness into conversations, I identified three qualities of mindful communication: calm, commitment, and curiosity. Let's look at each of these in turn to see how they can be woven into conversations.

Calm

Calm is the ability to stay grounded even when the conversation becomes emotional or difficult. When I think back on many of the conversations I had with my mother when I was younger, I am still struck by how often we would end up yelling at each other. We weren't necessarily angry; we would simply get very agitated. The energy would escalate, and before we knew it, we were yelling.

When you model calmness in conversation, the person you are talking to will give themselves more permission to consider their words and take their time. If they are not observing any agitation or impatience in you, they will likely have an easier time making their point and addressing everything on their mind. Disagreements are easier to deal with if you can remain steady and nonreactive.

We can achieve calm in conversation by remembering to breathe and by staying aware of our physical sensations. A very useful instruction I received many years ago from Frank Ostaseski was to keep about 30 percent of my attention in my body when talking with someone. This will support you to stay present to the conversation without getting lost in what is being said or becoming distracted. I have found that this practice also helps me stay committed to the conversation. It is a way of honoring my own needs while listening deeply.

Commitment

Commitment is the willingness to really show up for conversation, even when it becomes difficult. Sometimes this takes real courage when you don't know where the conversation will take you. Ultimately, you have to decide how much time you have to talk. If you have only a few minutes, you are not going to have a very deep conversation. I have found it helpful to set expectations before you begin a conversation by being very clear on how much time you have. If you have a few minutes, commit to being fully present for those minutes.

We express our commitment by our posture when in conversation. Standing sends a message that you are moving on as soon as you can. If you must stand because you have only a moment or two, acknowledge why you will remain standing. Again, this sets expectations. When you have time to sit, do you lean in or recline? Each posture sends a different message. Leaning in can feel to some people like there is anticipation or need. Reclining can be a sign that you are not taking what is being said seriously. Sitting upright in a neutral posture, if comfortable, conveys stability without signaling that you are expecting or resisting anything.

If you are caring for someone living with a serious illness, it may be difficult for them to express what they are thinking. I have noticed that for people living with serious illness, taking a long pause does not necessarily mean they are finished talking. We show our commitment by our willingness to relax into such silent pauses and wait to see if anything else is shared. Silence in conversation can feel very awkward. Notice if you are inclined to fill silence with your own words. See if instead you can sit quietly and wait. I have been amazed by what is expressed if we leave enough space for someone to muster the courage or energy to share something important.

Part of communicating with commitment is ending a conversation in a way that minimizes any unfinished business. I have found it useful to ask if what I have said is clear, or to say that we will need to finish the conversation later if it feels unfinished. I have often asked if there is anything else to talk about at the moment or to return to later. If it feels natural, you can thank the person you have been talking to for everything they have shared. This simple gesture conveys that what they shared matters to you.

Curiosity

Expressing curiosity about what the other person thinks or feels is an essential way to convey that you care about them. The most obvious way to express curiosity is to ask questions. Open-ended questions instead of questions that can be answered with a yes or a no deepen conversation.

In his seminal book on Zen practice, *Zen Mind, Beginner's Mind,*

Shunryu Suzuki, the founder of the San Francisco Zen Center, writes, "In the beginner's mind, there are many possibilities, but in the expert's mind there are few." Beginner's mind, or don't-know mind, is the ultimate expression of curiosity. Assuming this mindset invites us to question what we usually assume to be true. It is often difficult for family caregivers to apply a beginner's mindset when it comes to a loved one they have known for so many years. Whether or not you are caring for a family member, your bias about the person you are caring for may be very strong. It is very natural to hold certain assumptions about someone based on their past behavior or statements. I find it useful to ask myself the question, "How attached am I to this person behaving in a way that is consistent with what I know about them?"

Yes, you may know a lot about the person you are communicating with; however, can you set aside any assumptions you have about them and express curiosity as if you are meeting them for the first time? Living with an illness changes a person. Approaching a conversation with curiosity allows the person you are caring for to stay current with the realities of their present-moment circumstances. Your beginner's mind supports them to accept the changes their illness is imposing on them. When we resist the changes that illness brings, we add to our suffering. As a caregiver, you can help minimize that suffering by letting the person you care for be who they are in the moment. You do this by being aware of and letting go of your biases.

Staying for One More Breath

Communicating with the person you are caring for can present unique challenges. Even with the best intentions, it is easy to be misunderstood or to get triggered emotionally when in conversation. In chapter 4, I introduced Marilyn, with whom I sit regularly to offer emotional support. Her illness causes her extreme chronic pain. She often shares intense stories of her physical and emotional suffering, both her current challenges and her childhood trauma. While I view Marilyn's storytelling as a healthy outlet for her to process what she is experiencing, it can be very difficult to bear witness to her intense suffering. During some visits with her, I notice my strong desire to get up and leave, a reflection of my resistance to hearing about the pain she is sharing. And this is a natural response to hearing someone you care about express their suffering.

In these moments when I want to escape, I remind myself to stay in touch with my breath. Once I regain awareness of the breath, I tell myself that I can stay where I am. I can stay for one more breath and then another, and so on. Though I have learned that my companionship does make Marilyn feel better, it is not my job to make her feel better. My only job is to stay and offer a listening ear. In these moments, I recommit to staying present to whatever she shares.

Once I have regained a state of calm and have recommitted to staying, I find it easier to ask questions to keep her talking. My curiosity seems to send a message not only that I care but that I am paying attention to her words. Spending time with Marilyn requires a certain amount of creativity on my part. I think this is part of being curious. I look for something new I can ask her that may lead her to recognize her own resilience or to find meaning in her suffering.

Sadly, Marilyn has told me she doesn't have anyone else in her life who listens to her the way I do. What I do with her is so basic, yet for others in her life, it clearly does not come naturally. Her partner, her caregivers, and her friends grow impatient with her. It is not that what I do is all that special. For the ninety minutes I spend with her every other week, I make Marilyn the focus of my attention. Admittedly, this is made easier by the fact that I just drop in for a visit and leave when our time is up. I am not with Marilyn all day long, day after day, and she is not a family member with whom I have a long, complicated history. If you are caring for someone you are with constantly, offering curiosity in conversation will be especially difficult but still extremely beneficial.

Be really clear with yourself about what kind of conversation you want and how much energy you have. If you are pressed for time, again, be clear with the person you are talking with about how much time you have to offer them. When you need to leave, offer some kind of closure, and go. This is a healthy boundary to maintain. Most people like knowing exactly how much time they will have for a conversation. With Marilyn, I set a timer, which I do both for me and for her. If I am not honest with myself and her about how much time I have, I won't be able to stay present. Instead, I will begin thinking of ways to end the conversation, and that is not how I want to be with her.

You Don't Need to Know the Right Thing to Say

Weaving mindfulness into conversations allows you to let go of needing to know how a conversation is going to go. And mindful communication relieves you of having to know the right thing to say. Though it may feel counterintuitive, what is said is low on the list of what makes for a conversation that brings two people closer. When you converse with calm, commitment, and curiosity, your words matter less than your presence. As the poet Maya Angelou once said, "People will forget what you said, people will forget what you did, but people will never forget how you made them feel." Integrating mindfulness into your communications will make the people you interact with feel seen, connected, and cared for.

[Practice]

- Choose one quality of mindful communication — calm, commitment, or curiosity — and set an intention to apply the quality into one interaction. Afterward, when you have a quiet moment, review the experience and notice what effect your intention had on your conversation.
- Write in your journal what each of the qualities of mindful communication looks like for you.
- Try expanding your intention so that you bring more than one quality to your daily interactions.

CHAPTER 8

The Joy of Daily Practice

Every action, every gesture
An opportunity to strengthen my practice
Coming back to this precious moment

As a caregiver, you are busy and may not have extra time to devote to taking on a new and demanding routine. In this chapter we will look at several simple ways to train your mind by integrating into your daily routine what you have learned so far about mindfulness.

In one of our recent Mindful Caregiving Education classes, Maia shared her dismay at how often she and her mother, who she is caring for, end up arguing. Maia sees herself as wired to move quickly, and she gets frustrated when her mother can't keep up or disagrees with her. Maia didn't think it was possible to learn how to slow down and maintain mindful awareness. I have found this belief to be quite common. I told Maia what I tell other caregivers who don't see a way out of their reactive patterns: I suggested she start with simple mindfulness interventions that would help her pause and return to the present moment. I explained that starting small and practicing would give her new habits that would begin to feel automatic. Simplifying the practice is the easiest way to develop skills that bring a sense of ease and build emotional resilience.

Even if you see yourself as wired like Maia — easily taken into states of impatience or frustration — you can also easily enter into a state of complete presence. Think about moments when you have been absorbed by some activity or something in your environment. Hearing the sound of a songbird. Seeing a stunning sunset. Witnessing delight expressed by a young child. Tasting the first bite of a delicious meal. In these moments, you are not consciously setting an intention to be fully aware of what is happening; you are just transported there without even thinking about it. As you practice daily, you will begin to notice that it takes less and less effort to move into and maintain mindful awareness. You will be training your mind to return to present-moment awareness with ease. At first, however, it will require a commitment to practice.

Mindfulness practice does not need to be overly complicated. Although meditation is the best way to learn mindfulness, you do not need to sit quietly with your legs crossed on a cushion for thirty minutes a day to practice. You don't need to buy a meditation cushion and a bell and find an appropriate quiet spot in your home to meditate. If you did do these things, that would be wonderful, and you would probably acquire mindfulness skills more quickly. However, formal meditation is not absolutely necessary to build mindfulness skills. The beauty of mindfulness is that you can use many of your current activities to learn how to achieve and maintain present-moment awareness and calm.

You will reap the most benefit if you use every opportunity to practice. The more you practice, the faster you will notice results. People progress at different rates, and you may feel like it is taking a long time to notice any change in how you respond to stress or difficult situations. Trust is an important part of learning these ancient mindfulness techniques, lending you the permission and the encouragement to try them. I always tell caregivers to take on mindfulness practice as a thought experiment. Try it for a while and see if you notice anything different in how you feel and behave. If this is sounding like a lot of work, I assure you that taking on a practice is actually quite simple, and you will probably enjoy the momentary experiences of engaging mindful awareness.

Let's look at using tasks you already engage in as opportunities to deepen your mindfulness practice. Take a moment to contemplate a caregiving activity that you engage in regularly. It could be as simple as washing dishes or folding laundry. Imagine yourself going through the motions of the task. Give your full attention to the different movements associated with the task. Think of every sensation you might experience as you carry out the activity. What do your hands feel? What smells do you notice? What sounds are part of the activity? What are you looking at as you perform the task? What motions are necessary to complete the task? If distracting thoughts arise as you recall the activity, see if you can let go of the thoughts and return to imagining yourself engaging in the task. Try this for a few moments before reading on.

The way you just practiced, paying careful attention to the moment-to-moment details of a particular task, is how you strengthen your ability to focus your attention. While engaged in an activity, you should still be able to notice if you become distracted by thoughts unrelated to the activity. As you have been learning, this is about direct experience, noticing the engagement of the five senses. Such attention to detail is not about what happened before or what will happen next; it is about staying in the present moment with the full sensory experience. Is there anything about your experience of this activity that you have never noticed before?

Now that you have practiced careful awareness in action by recalling a common activity you engage in, you are ready to try it in real time. The next time you put down this book, try applying mindful awareness to whatever activity you move into. As we have discussed, the key is to keep coming back to direct experience. Notice when you get distracted by thoughts or disruptions in your environment, let go of the distractions, and come back to full engagement in your activity.

Resetting Your Mind

Let's turn to some practices you can engage in throughout your day that will support you in resetting your mind when you are feeling overwhelmed or stressed. These are simple but effective. Before you know it, you will use these techniques without really giving them much thought. Try them all, and see which ones feel the most natural. Before you know it, you will have your favorites.

Touching the Door Frame

When entering the room or home of the person you are caring for, pause at the entryway. You might place a hand on the door frame and check in with your physical sensations, your emotions, or your thoughts. You can ask yourself, "What am I carrying into this encounter?" Use this moment to let go of whatever you do not need or whatever may make your encounter difficult. Use the pause to reset your mind to present-moment awareness. Then, when you are ready, step in.

Shaking It Out

To symbolically let go of thoughts or emotions that may be unhelpful, you might set down whatever object you are holding and shake out your hands. Tell yourself you are letting go of whatever is not useful or needed.

Planted Feet

You can pause at any time to feel your feet in contact with the ground. As you notice the sensations of your feet, remember that you are in contact with the ground. You might remind yourself that this solid earth holds and supports your experience.

Hand on Your Chest

Wherever you are, whatever you are doing, you can always place a hand on your chest over your heart. Notice the sensations of this contact between your hand and your chest. Can you feel your heartbeat? If your thoughts spin off into a story about what you are feeling, try to come back to noticing sensations. Rest here for a few breaths, and then move on to whatever is calling your attention next.

Attentive Drinking

When taking a break to have a drink of water, tea, coffee, and so on, give your full attention to the sensations of drinking. What sensations associated with drinking have you not noticed before? What do you notice about the temperature of the liquid? How about its thickness? What flavors do you notice? When you swallow, how far into your throat do you notice sensation? What do you notice about the texture of the cup or glass you are holding? Who knew there was so much to notice about the simple act of taking a drink? You can also apply this kind of attention to eating.

One with the Soundscape

When possible, step outdoors and find a safe place to close your eyes. Take in the soundscape around you. Try to keep your attention on the sensation of hearing without needing to identify the sounds you hear. You are not listening to understand or find meaning; you are simply letting the sounds come to you as they are. If judgment about a particular sound arises, try to let it go. Let yourself rest in the soundscape, just as it is.

Expansive Awareness

When you are feeling emotional or physical discomfort, expanding your awareness beyond the body can be supportive. Emotional and physical pain can cause you to contract your awareness, contributing to a feeling of being confined in current circumstances. Expanding your awareness can remind you of the larger context of your experience, and this can bring a more expansive perspective and even comfort.

Begin by attuning to your immediate surroundings. Then begin to expand outward. How far do your eyes see? What are the farthest edges of your hearing? Make sure you stay with what is true to your sensory experience. As soon as your imagination is activated, return to direct experience. When uncomfortable sensations or emotions arise, do your best to return your focus to the outer edges of your present-moment awareness. Let this expanded awareness remind you of the much larger world that is holding your experience of discomfort.

STOP Practice

The STOP practice is very easy to remember and use. When you find yourself in a difficult situation, or when your mind is on overdrive, simply *Stop*. This momentary pause from what you are doing or thinking can change everything. You are catching yourself, coming back into self-reflection or awareness. It may be easier to think of this first step as returning to inner stillness. When circumstances demand that you stay on the task at hand, returning to inner stillness in the midst of action is an expression of grace.

After stopping, *Take a breath*, and then another. Spend a moment or two focusing on your inhalation and exhalation, just as you've learned in previous chapters. This step brings you back into the body, back into the sensing mind and present-moment awareness.

Once you have returned to present-moment awareness by stopping and taking a breath, *Observe* your experience. Notice what is happening with sensations, emotions, and thoughts as you meet your current situation. What is happening with those you encounter? What stories are you telling yourself about the situation or encounter? This is an opportunity to plan your response or shift your attitude, a chance to recalibrate and begin again.

The final step is to *Proceed* with whatever you were doing when you stopped. You can choose to proceed in a way that supports you and others as you show up as your best self. How you choose to proceed may deescalate a challenging encounter or offer a new perspective on a difficult situation.

Breath Awareness

Breath awareness at its core is very basic, yet there are many different ways of attuning to the breath. Here are a few techniques for making the breath a safe refuge from a chaotic situation or an agitated mind.

Counting

Counting your breaths is a great way to begin. Count each breath as you exhale. See if you can count up to five breaths, and then begin again at one. If you become distracted and lose count, no problem, simply begin again at one. Once you reach a count of five, begin again at one.

Labeling

Labeling your inhale and exhale is an easy way to keep your attention focused on the breath. As you exhale, silently say to yourself, "Exhale." As you inhale, silently say to yourself, "Inhale." You can say, "Breathing in" and "Breathing out." Say whatever feels natural to you.

Sometimes I will repeat silently to myself, "On the inhale I come back...on the exhale I let go." Or "On the inhale I notice...on the exhale I let go." You can find your own ways to use inhaling and exhaling to maintain your focus.

Box Breathing

Box breathing is slightly more complicated but extremely effective for anchoring your attention on the breath. Beginning with the inhale, you slowly breathe in for a length of time that is comfortable for you, and then you hold your breath for another few seconds before exhaling. Then you exhale slowly for as long as you find comfortable and again pause for a few seconds before inhaling again. You might start with a four-second inhale, followed by a four-second pause. Then exhale for four seconds, followed by a four-second pause. It may take you two or three breaths before you find a comfortable rhythm.

Attuning to Sensations of the Breath

Finally, you can simply attune to the sensations associated with breathing in and breathing out, as introduced in chapter 3. How curious can you be about what is happening in the body as you breathe in and breathe out? What do you notice? When your thoughts drift away from the sensations you notice, let go of the distracting thoughts and come back.

These practices will build your capacity to be with whatever shows up on your path. The process of training your mind allows you to be with what is actually happening without denying or masking your authentic experience. Your body craves your attention. Attuning to your body and its myriad sensations brings you back to a state of wholeness. It is in this state of intimacy and integration that healing takes place. Although everyone's body and mind will eventually cause problems and distress, the body and mind are worthy of boundless appreciation and attention. Learning to attune to your physical and emotional experience will enhance your well-being. When you feel better, your caregiving shows it, and the person you are caring for feels it.

[Practice]

Participants in Zen Caregiving Project courses consistently find the STOP practice to be a memorable and highly effective technique for mental reset. It's an invaluable tool, easily recalled and applied even in moments of intense agitation.

- Throughout your day, use the STOP practice when you notice you are feeling even the slightest agitation. It may be difficult to remember to use the STOP practice when agitation arises or when you find yourself in a stressful situation, but it will become more natural over time as you practice.
- At first you might consider setting an alarm as a reminder to apply the STOP practice a few times during your day.
- Note in your journal any changes you notice in how you deal with stressful situations when applying the STOP practice. Or record what gets in the way of using the practice.
- Consider introducing the person you are caring for to the STOP practice. Once they are familiar with the four steps, look for opportunities to invite them to use the practice, such as during disagreements, when you notice their agitation, or when a reset is needed.

COMPASSION

Compassion is not a relationship between healer and the wounded.
It is a relationship between equals.

— Pema Chödrön

We do good because it frees the heart.
It opens us to a wellspring of happiness.

— Sharon Salzberg

CHAPTER 9

Redefining Compassion

With this quivering heart
I awaken to the suffering around me
Courage leads me to action
Serving others as I serve myself

[**Compassion can be broken down into five distinct stages. Understanding each stage will help you recognize where you get stuck. In this chapter we will define *compassion* and begin looking at its role in caregiving.**]

Late one night, I was on a train returning home after a caregiving shift. I was tired but happy and looking forward to arriving home. The train car was sparsely filled with passengers. We pulled into a station, and I watched the doors slide open. As an older man exited the train, something slid from his pocket and dropped to the floor. Without thinking, I jumped up, picked up the plastic card, and ran off the train to catch the man. I returned the card to him, telling him he had dropped it. I turned around and was able to reenter the train just as the doors were closing. I remember sitting back down and being surprised at how quickly the event took place. I noticed I had an expansive sense of ease and gratification.

When looking back on that night, I am moved by how readily my hospice shift flowed into the rest of my life. My inclination to do something to address the suffering of another could not be confined to the place I knew as "hospice." We are all dying, so why would I treat a stranger walking down the street differently than I would a patient living their final days in hospice? The way I acted to lessen the suffering of the man getting off the train was nothing special; acting compassionately toward others is a basic human attribute. I know this to be true, yet the action that night also somehow felt significant. It reminded me of how I wanted to be in the world.

Compassion in Common

Something I find unfortunate about writing this book and putting it out into the world is that very likely it will not be possible for me to know you, the reader. Like the caregivers I meet regularly, I want to sit with you and hear the story of your caregiving experience. Although we have not met, I am certain we have things in common. We both want to be happy. We both want to be free from unnecessary suffering. And we are both compassionate beings. You would not be a caregiver if you were not a compassionate person. These are the things I know about you.

Each of us is brought into the world with the inclination to act compassionately programmed into our being. If this were not true, we as a species would never have survived for as long as we have. And yet, due to early traumas and negative conditioning, some of us lose the inclination to act compassionately. The good news is that relearning and strengthening compassion is always within our reach.

What is compassion? Every spiritual tradition around the world teaches about compassion as an expression of both our innate goodness and our oneness with other beings. In Latin, *passio*, or passion, means "to suffer," "to endure," or "to bear." The prefix *com* means "with." So, in a Judeo-Christian sense, compassion means "to suffer with." In the Jewish Old Testament, God commands the Israelites to be compassionate, even to their enemies. In the book of Peter in the New Testament, "gentle Christians" are instructed to love one another and to be compassionate. In Buddhist philosophy, the *brahmaviharas*, the four heavenly abodes, are foundational teachings. One abode is *karuna*, the

Pali word for compassion, meaning the desire to reduce the suffering of others. Throughout the holy text of Islam, the Quran, we find references to *rahmah*, which is translated as "mercy" or "compassion." Compassion is universal. It is essentially human.

Given the direct relationship between compassion and suffering, it may be useful to offer a working definition of *suffering*, which can imply different things depending on your background. I have come to view suffering as simply wanting things to be different from how they are. To be human means we suffer. There is no way around this. If you are living with a serious debilitating illness, your suffering will likely be profound and obvious. However, even small discomforts or obstacles in healthy people can cause a lot of suffering if they strongly resist the experience of things not being the way they want them to be. And suffering is addressed by compassion.

Compassion Is Caregiving

The role of compassion in caregiving is central. Even if you feel you do not have a choice in taking on the role of caregiver, if you weren't compassionate, you would find a way to avoid the responsibility. We all hear stories of abandonment and neglect; however, you have chosen another path. Though compassion motivates you to care for another, it is natural for compassion to get blocked from time to time, and you may not always feel compassionate. Blocked compassion can make your caregiving feel extremely burdensome. In later chapters we will examine the ways in which compassion gets blocked and ways to overcome it.

Historically, compassion has been understood in the context of spirituality, yet recently a growing number of scientific studies have been devoted to researching what happens in the brain when we experience compassion. Current scientific research supports what spiritual traditions have been teaching for ages, that the experience of compassion and kindness makes us feel better about ourselves and the world around us.

Five Stages of Compassion

When I was studying to become a teacher of Compassion Cultivation Training, a program developed at Stanford University, I learned that the dynamic process of experiencing compassion consists of five distinct steps. Understanding each of these steps will help you recognize why you feel compassion when you do, and where at other times you get stuck. Let's look at each step.

Awareness

First, there must be an awareness of suffering. The entire first part of this book explored awareness, so you know that distraction is common and can prevent you from seeing what is happening within and around you. I live in the San Francisco Bay Area, and as in many parts of the country, we see a lot of people living on the streets here. This societal problem can feel overwhelming. The suffering of people without a home is front and center in many neighborhoods, yet if I choose to look away, I can ignore it.

In your caregiving role, there are likely things you do not notice. If you are caring for someone who is nonverbal, they may convey their discomfort through facial expressions or their body language, yet if you are not watching them, you will not see that they are uncomfortable. The first step of experiencing compassion is to notice suffering wherever it shows up.

Empathy

For most of us, when we are confronted with the suffering of another, we will experience a visceral response. This is the empathic stage of compassion. You are human, so you know what it means to be in physical pain or to be emotionally overwhelmed. Because you know, you can empathize with another person's challenging experience. You probably recall times when you saw someone get injured and you cringed. This is the pain-processing center of the brain sending messages to the body. You will remember the explanation in chapter 6 about mirror neurons in regard to emotions, but mirror neurons also get activated when we witness physical pain in another. This brain activity is what happens when we have an empathic response to suffering. Keep in mind that empathy is activated not only by negative emotions or pain but also by witnessing positive emotions.

Empathy and compassion are not the same. Empathy feeds compassion. It is essential for compassion, but it is not the same as compassion. If you stop at this second stage of compassion when you see suffering, you are not truly expressing compassion. Stopping at this stage without giving your empathy an outlet through compassionate action can result in negative feelings, stress, and even physical problems. This will be discussed more fully when we talk about barriers to compassion.

Intention

The empathic response is typically followed by a desire to see suffering reduced. This is the intentional stage. This inclination is your essential goodness and your deep knowing that we are all in this together being expressed. Yes, we are individuals; however, we are all connected in the common experience of being human, with all its joys and struggles. Even if you are not able to stop and do something in the moment, you will likely experience thoughts about how the suffering can be addressed, or you will feel an activation in your body that signifies a readiness to do something. Although this stage is important and noble, it too is not exactly compassion.

Action

In order for compassion to be genuinely expressed, some action must follow your intention to alleviate suffering. If you do not take action to address the suffering you see, you are not truly showing compassion. It is easy to hold certain assumptions about what the action must look like, and this is where I believe a lot of people get confused.

The story a caregiver named Annalee shared about her mother illustrates the point that compassionate action does not always look the way we think it should. Annalee shared that her mother raised four daughters on her own and had always been very independent and strong. Due to the progression of her illness, Annalee's mother had to learn to let others help her; however, it has not been easy.

Annalee's mother is in charge of her own medications. After a recent medical procedure, she was left with pain and needed to keep on top of it with medication. Annalee learned that her mother does not like to be reminded to take her meds. If she encourages her mother to take pain medication before she begins to feel pain, her mother becomes angry.

One afternoon she saw that her mother was showing signs of being in pain. Of course, Annalee wanted to tell her mom to take her meds. Instead, recognizing how important it is for her mother to feel in control, Annalee said nothing, even though she knew her mom would suffer. And, being late to act on the pain, her mother became extremely uncomfortable before the pain meds began working.

Since then, Annalee's mother has admitted that she forgets to take the medication when she is not experiencing pain and requested help with remembering. Annalee set an alarm on both their phones at the times when the medication needs to be taken. Sometimes, the compassionate action is to let someone you care about learn in their own time what you already know, even if that leaves them suffering in some way. (Obviously, this does not pertain to when such suffering could be life-threatening.)

Compassionate action does not always look like action. Consider this situation. Someone is extremely ill and in pain. They have requested more pain medication, and it has been given, but it has not yet relieved the pain. The most you may be able to do is to sit quietly and hold a hand or stroke a shoulder. Your commitment to being present with them is an extremely compassionate act, even though it may not feel like you are doing much.

Compassionate action in response to another's suffering is not always directed at the person whose suffering you are aware of. For instance, when you find yourself in a situation where you believe you need to let the person suffering learn their own lessons, or you want to act but others are on the scene tending to the person, the most you may be able to do is to address your own suffering with compassionate action. Not acting to alleviate another's suffering can be emotionally painful, whether it is due to your decision or to circumstances. In these moments, self-compassion is the most skillful outlet for your inclination to do something. We will look more closely at self-compassion in chapter 12.

Warm Glow

Finally, when we move through each step of compassion, and we alleviate someone else's suffering, we experience a positive feeling. The reward centers of the brain are activated, leaving us with a feeling that is referred to as the "warm glow." Can you think of a time when you did something for someone else and it left you feeling this warm glow?

It may feel a bit strange to dwell in the warm glow and celebrate yourself for acting compassionately, but we know that it is very healthy to experience this sensation, since it reinforces compassion. If there was no reward, you may not be as inclined to act compassionately in the future. It is not selfish or indulgent to let yourself fully experience the warm glow. The world needs more compassion, so let yourself enjoy the good feeling that comes with showing up with an open heart and taking action for others.

[Practice]

- The next time you do something to address another person's suffering, see if afterward you can identify the five distinct stages of compassion you experienced.
- Remember, your act of compassion does not need to be some grand gesture. Don't overlook the beauty of simply treating someone kindly and offering a smile. Just conveying to someone who appears lonely that you see them can be an enormous act of compassion. How does acting with compassion make you feel?

CHAPTER 10

Becoming a Compassionate Companion

May I move toward the suffering
I see around me
Let my words and actions
Transform suffering into love

Suffering is part of the human experience, and no one is immune. In this chapter, we look more closely at compassion's central role in addressing the suffering of people who need the support of others.

Suffering arises from the changes time inevitably brings. There are four significant human stages of life referred to as the *heavenly messengers* in Buddhist teachings: birth, old age, sickness, and death. Each of us is born, and each of us will die. Most of us will experience old age, and most of us will experience sickness. These "messengers" are an inevitable part of being human. The message that each of these life stages carry is that everything changes, everything is impermanent.

The person you are caring for is having their turn. It is their time for sickness. Or maybe they have reached old age. Or perhaps the end of their life has arrived. We each take our turn experiencing such events. Your turn will come. When it is your turn to suffer through difficult events that bring significant change, you will have your unique way of dealing with the reality of your circumstances. You may be able to meet old age, sickness, and death with ease and joy, but probably not continuously. You may be just as scared, resistant, controlling, complaining, impatient, demanding, or stubborn as the person you are caring for. Most of us will at some point share our misery with those around us.

Having a companion along for the journey when it is our turn to face difficulty is a blessing. Facing a major challenge like old age, sickness, or death is a lonely business. Living with a chronic illness that flares up from time to time, I know how isolating the experience of illness can be. You don't have the energy to be with or even reach out to friends or family. You feel so crappy, you may push people away. You feel as though others cannot imagine what you are going through, or you feel shame about how you look or feel. Others may feel awkward around you, so they avoid you. In these cases, human contact is actually a gift, a gift that often comes in the form of a caregiver. When as caregivers we recognize that suffering is universal and that sooner or later we too will suffer, we have an easier time meeting the person we care for in their suffering.

Reciprocity of Serving Others

When I trained to become a caregiver at Zen Hospice Project, I learned to view caregiving as "serving" others rather than "helping." Though the distinction may seem unimportant, when we care for others with compassion, we are conveying that we are no better and no worse than them. *Helping* conveys the sense that the one we support is missing something and that we are providing that missing piece. It can imply that the person we are caring for is somehow less complete than we are.

Serving others is about expressing our deepest truth about being human. Serving recognizes our sameness and the reciprocity that is inherent in offering care. I am convinced it is impossible to offer care without getting something in return. I am not referring to some form of material compensation but to the warm glow mentioned in the last chapter, as well as a sense of purpose, lessons about what it means to suffer as a human, and the pure pleasure of connecting deeply with another person.

It is impossible to care for others without growing or evolving as a human being. Often I have entered into a caregiving relationship thinking I was there to give something back, and yet I always feel I have received so much more from the experience than the person I was supporting. In a favorite Zen story, a young monk approaches his teacher and asks, "Teacher, how do I serve others?" The teacher replies, "Forget about serving others, serve yourself." Slightly confused, the monk asks, "How do I serve myself?" The old teacher then says, "Forget about serving yourself, serve others."

This story reminds me that serving myself and serving others are tightly woven together. What is truly good for me is good for others, and what is good for others is good for me. As humans, we are all in this together. When you show up as a caregiver with mindful awareness, that is, without all the thoughts that contribute to feeling separate from others, there is really no difference between you and those you serve. Of course, there are circumstantial differences; the person you care for is likely living with some kind of illness or does not have the physical or emotional strength to carry on without the support of others, and you do not need the same kind of support. And while you may be in the role of caregiver today, sooner or later, as noted above, you will also need care. In this sense, there is really no difference between you and the person you care for. We can meet each other in our mutual vulnerability as humans who suffer.

Surrendering to Circumstances

Apart from circumstantial differences, something that varies from person to person is how they deal with discomfort and difficulty. Perhaps you have heard the saying "Pain is inevitable, but suffering is optional." I came to really understand this when I met Adrian, who died at the guest house facility. As she approached her death, her body went through the familiar changes. She lost weight. She grew weaker to the point where she could no longer get out of bed. Her skin began to break down. Her body was failing her. And through it all she was quite open with her family and with our staff and volunteers about what was happening. She knew she was dying and faced it without turning away. What was remarkable was that despite her discomforts, she seemed to be suffering very little. She discovered newfound joy in the little things she could still do and see. Adrian loved the colorful fabrics her daughter brought her to use as head wraps. She took delight in the flowers delivered to her room. She smiled at the soft music filling the space around her. Adrian was able to drop all resistance. She was at peace with what was happening. In my observation, she had moved into complete surrender to her experience. She was happy, calm, and very present.

Adrian was extraordinary, and she was no different from any of us. Although we each have the potential to reach a place of complete surrender to our circumstances, in all my years of witnessing people approaching their death or living with long-term illness, it has been rare to meet someone experiencing that level of peace and ease. More often than not, patients living with serious illness are very resistant to what is happening. This does not make them bad people, weak, or lazy; it is just how they end up meeting their situation after years of conditioning, trauma, and habits. No one wants to live with a serious illness, but when it happens, that is what is happening; it is what life becomes. And the more we resist, the more we suffer.

The Second Arrow

A Zen teaching that I have found helpful in understanding how we create unnecessary suffering is the analogy of the "second arrow." There is the first arrow, the situation that causes pain or inconvenience. The first arrow is what it is. However, so many people meet the situation with resistance. They may fret that the pain will worsen, think unkind things about how they caused the situation, focus on all the ways they could have avoided the situation, look for someone or something to blame for the pain. All this mental churning is the second arrow. This is the suffering we bring on by being stuck in our thoughts. I think it is helpful to remember that when driving down the highway, walking down the aisle at the grocery store, or stepping into the home of someone who is ill, many arrows are flying through the air.

Responding to the suffering of another with compassion is an expression of what I heard the Zen teacher Roshi Bernie Glassman call an "expanded sense of self." Roshi Bernie was known to have said, "May we always have the courage to bear witness, to see ourselves as others and to see others as ourselves." When another suffers, we suffer too. This is easy to understand when you witness the suffering of someone close to you. When my wife is ill, I feel bad about it. When I think about the suffering my father experiences as he grows older, I feel directly impacted.

Limitless Suffering

Yet suffering knows no limits. It is not limited to only those you care about. It may not be as easy to fully acknowledge the suffering of people you don't know or don't care about as it is with those you love. However, you only need to turn on the news, open a newspaper, or walk down a street in any city or small town to see suffering around you. The suffering in the world also has an impact on your sense of well-being in both subtle and profound ways. Even the suffering of those in "outside groups" is not separate from any of us. Martin Luther King Jr. offered this idea of shared suffering when he wrote, "Injustice anywhere is a threat to justice everywhere. We are caught in an inescapable network of mutuality, tied in a single garment of destiny. Whatever affects one directly, affects all indirectly." The good news is that human compassion, when expressed, knows no limits.

Bottomless Well of Compassion

Despite your best intentions, you may at times believe the suffering of the person you care for is more than you can handle. This thinking imposes an artificial limitation on your compassion. Your experience of exhaustion, overwhelm, and sadness are very real, no doubt about it; however, you also possess a bottomless well of compassion. Your ability to access this compassion determines your capacity to be with the suffering of others. The question becomes, Can you access these depths of compassion?

Accessing compassion is not always easy. It is common for all sorts of barriers to get in the way, and we will explore some of them in chapter 13. For now let's just acknowledge that sometimes what gets in the way of expressing compassion for others is a focus on oneself. Many of us are raised to focus on taking care of our own needs without asking for or offering help. Speaking for myself, I spent much of my life with a "me-first" attitude. My inclination to support others, which I believe we are each born with, was largely supplanted by external messaging that convinced me that I should only look out for myself.

Expressing compassion has the emotional effect of naturally shifting our focus away from self and onto others. In other words, the more we cultivate compassion, the easier it becomes to notice and respond to the suffering around us. You may think that paying more attention to the suffering around you will become burdensome, depressing, or even harmful. This assumption is quite common. I have stopped counting the number of times someone has suggested to me that working with chronically or seriously ill people must be really hard or depressing. However, I have found the opposite to be true. Genuine compassion provides a kind of immunity from the emotional heaviness of bearing witness to suffering. This is because genuine compassion always includes an action, a practical outlet for emotions, and will almost always lead to positive feelings of warmth and fulfillment.

If suffering is an inevitable part of being human, and if each of us has a bottomless well of compassion, why is it that we live in a society in which there seems to be such a shortage of compassion? If more people were conversant in how compassion works, maybe things would be different. Wouldn't it be amazing if compassion was a primary school subject like math, science, and history and was taught in every primary school in the world? Although I am certain this would change our world for the better, compassion is rarely taught in school. So I am not surprised when I often encounter confusion around what compassion is. Let's address any confusion by first looking at what compassion is *not.*

- Compassion is not pity. Pity is the experience of sorrow over another person's suffering or misfortune without the inclination to do anything to address the suffering. Pity is based on an assumption of being different from the person who suffers rather than seeing their vulnerability as no different from your own. Pity is seeing suffering but not doing anything to alleviate it.
- Compassion is not the personal distress you may feel when you see another person suffering. This distress is the result of overidentifying with the suffering you witness and being unable to channel your empathic concern into genuine compassionate action.
- Compassion is not a sign of weakness. In fact, compassion often requires courage and can look fierce. Just think of a parent who protects their child from a threat.
- Compassion is not the sense of relief that at least you are not the one experiencing the difficulty.
- Compassion is not denying another person's experience of suffering under the guise of tough love. Compassion acknowledges another person's suffering even if you would not suffer under the same circumstances.
- Compassion is not necessarily heroism, even though a heroic act could be what you extend to alleviate the suffering you witness.
- Compassion does not have to entail a personal sacrifice, although it may take that form.

Now let's take another look at what compassion is. Compassion is an expression of humanity's highest potential. It conveys the beauty and wonder of an open heart. Being a companion to someone who struggles with a health challenge is one of life's noblest endeavors, and it can at times be impossibly difficult. Yet the way you offer care to others defines who you are and the world you would like to see. It also demonstrates to others how you would like to be treated when you are at your most vulnerable. One thing each of us can count on is that sooner or later we too will be at our most vulnerable and will require the care of a compassionate companion.

[Practice]

In this practice activity, work with noticing how open you are to seeing the suffering of the person you are caring for.

- Using what you have learned in previous chapters, maintain emotional steadiness when you are with the person you are caring for, and try to notice the subtle or obvious signs of how they are feeling.
- Notice if you are receptive to any signs of distress or if you avoid them.
- Does your heart open or close?
- Notice if you feel drawn in, aversion, or indifference.
- Try not to judge your response; just notice.
- Think about what gets in the way of noticing the suffering of the person you are caring for.

CHAPTER 11

Loving-Kindness

May I and all beings be happy
May I and all beings be safe and free from danger
May I and all beings be well
May I and all beings be at peace

While compassion is focused on suffering, loving-kindness is focused on well-being. They are the two sides of the same coin. In this chapter we will look at how generating and extending loving-kindness contributes to feelings of happiness and satisfaction.

Wishes for Well-Being

Take a moment as you begin this chapter to close your eyes and picture someone you care about. Choose a person with whom you have an uncomplicated relationship, perhaps an infant or a small child, a dear friend, or even an animal companion. Imagine this person or being sitting in front of you as you look into their eyes. Now silently extend wishes for their well-being. Send them wishes for comfort, ease, good health, abundance, and happiness. Try not to hold back. Send them as many wishes as you can think of. Let your warmth and goodness radiate out toward them. As you do this, notice how it makes you feel in your heart. Notice how it makes you feel generally. Stay with the visualization for as long as you like.

You've just experienced loving-kindness in action. Loving-kindness is the desire to see others experiencing ease and well-being. It differs from compassion in that compassion is focused on meeting and alleviating the suffering of another, while loving-kindness is the wish for another to experience joy, safety, and wellness. Like compassion, loving-kindness is also one of the four heavenly abodes introduced in chapter 9. Both reflect the goodness of an open heart and mind. Both are necessary components in a healthy and fulfilling life as a relational being. A note: The Pali term *metta* is typically translated as "loving-kindness" or "unconditional friendliness." In our discussion I will use the terms *kindness* and *loving-kindness.*

Loving-kindness, like compassion, can transform your caregiving. Others will sense your loving-kindness even when you do not use words to express your feelings. Think of someone who extended kindness to you. How did it feel to be in their presence? Was what you felt dependent on what they said? When we receive loving-kindness, it is a felt sensation; the body senses kindness in others. Receiving kindness from others expands and elevates our heart and mind.

Caregiving Is More Than Competency

For a caregiver it is natural and good to focus on doing things well. And while it is important to be competent in your caregiving, competency is not enough. The person receiving your competency without kindness will experience it as mechanical and objectifying. In other words, if you are only competent, the person receiving your care will be made to feel like an object and not fully human. Caregiving without kindness creates distance between you and the person you care for. Competency without kindness is better than nothing — but just barely.

I have seen how competent caregiving is received when loving-kindness is absent. Those receiving care may be appreciative, but they too become mechanical or even shut down. It is like they are simply trying to make it through the encounter. It can feel like the caregiver and the person receiving care are not even in the same room together. This is heartbreaking to witness and contributes to the isolation so many people living with illness experience.

Overcoming Obstacles to Kindness

I am certain most caregivers want to be warm and kind; however, time constraints often become a disruptive force. For many caregivers, busyness gets in the way of expressing from the heart. Even the kindest person cannot maintain active loving-kindness twenty-four hours a day. I love my family dearly, and I think most people who have met me would say I am a kind person, yet often I struggle to access loving-kindness and direct it toward others. Resentment, envy, biases, contempt, and other distracting thoughts interfere with the flow of loving-kindness. Only present-moment awareness will cut through the mind chatter that obstructs accessing the warm heart of loving-kindness.

The next time you feel you cannot access kindness toward the person you care for, find an opportunity to pause and notice what thoughts are getting in the way. Then remind yourself that just like you, the person you care for wants to be happy. They too have suffered. They too have hopes and dreams. Then try to drop into present-moment awareness for a moment or two. Disruptive thoughts may arise, but do your best not to feed them. Then begin to imagine that you are radiating warm light from your heart to the person you care for. With that warm light, extend wishes for their well-being, as you did in the contemplation at the start of this chapter. Send them wishes for comfort, ease, good health, abundance, and happiness. If extending kindness in this way feels inauthentic or awkward at first, give yourself permission to fake it. Over time it will become more natural.

When you try to awaken loving-kindness, you will likely notice that negative thoughts — about the person you care for specifically or about your life generally — are quite persistent. This is common. Do your best to use what you learned in part 1 of the book to maintain focus on extending loving-kindness outward.

Loving-Kindness Contributes to Happiness

As with compassionate action, the more you work to access loving-kindness and extend it to others, the better you will feel generally. Barbara Fredrickson, a professor of psychology at the University of North Carolina, studied the effects of a regular loving-kindness meditation, one similar to the contemplation at the beginning of the chapter. The study found that a regular practice of loving-kindness led to an increase in positive emotions and life satisfaction. Other studies have found similar results.

So far, we have considered extending loving-kindness to the person you are caring for or the people you care about. However, if extending kindness in these types of relationships is beneficial, why stop there? Understandably, it is much more difficult to extend kindness to people you find annoying, strangers, or people you perceive to be different from you. When you notice you have difficulty generating kindness for those who are part of "outside" groups, simply remind yourself that they too want to be happy. They too have hopes and dreams. They too have people in their lives whom they love and who love them.

In broadening the circle of your loving-kindness, it is also helpful to consider how intertwined your life is with the lives of complete strangers. It is not a stretch to say that your well-being depends on the lives and work of people you have never met. Thupten Jinpa makes a convincing case in his book *A Fearless Heart*, which explores the power of compassion to change lives:

> Take for example the various necessities of our life — the things we require to maintain our life and health and flourish. From the food we eat, the clothes we wear, and the home we live in to the books we enjoy reading, the ideas that inspire

> us, and the many services we take advantage of every day, we depend on others for every one of our comforts and joys… and for our very survival.

The practice of broadening your circle of loving-kindness is especially useful when the person you care for is not a family member or friend. A caregiver who attended one of our courses a few years back shared that the person she was caring for was very racist. This remarkable caregiver identified as BIPOC, and the man she cared for was an older white man who expressed distasteful views. She explained that at first she was very reactive to his off-handed comments. Nonetheless, needing the income, she returned each day. As time passed, she got to know the man a little better. She came to understand how the struggles in his life contributed to his attitudes toward people of color. She began to see how this had closed his heart. While she did not excuse his offensive behavior, and even called him out at times, she was able to extend kindness to him. She could see that the part of this man able to recognize the worthiness and beauty of all beings was broken. And her ability to recognize his brokenness allowed her to extend kindness toward him.

Constant external pressures work against our natural inclination toward loving-kindness. I often feel as though leaders in government, media, and even religious communities are trying desperately to convince us that people who are unlike us are somehow less than human and not worthy of our kindness. They seem to believe this will somehow benefit them. Too many in our society limit their loving-kindness to a small group of people. This kind of modern-day tribalism contributes to many of the problems we see around us, such as political division, discrimination, the normalization of hate speech, and even military action. I view caregivers as leaders in a movement to break down the barriers that separate us. Caregivers know better than anyone that we are all vulnerable and worthy of kindness. Even if you struggle to generate loving-kindness toward the person you care for, the act of caregiving is itself a choice for kindness, and that choice has the potential to change lives and society for the better.

[Practice]

One of my favorite activities that we facilitate as part of some of our in-person classes is what I call the loving-kindness walkabout. Participants walk around randomly within a designated space. At intervals, the group is asked to stop and look at someone in the group who is not looking back at them. Then they are guided to extend loving-kindness to the person they are looking at. Try the loving-kindness walkabout on your own.

- You can try this practice by walking around any space where others gather. It can be your neighborhood, a park, or a shopping mall. However, you can also do this sitting at home by imagining family members, friends, and even people in your neighborhood whom you see from time to time.
- Find or imagine someone to whom you direct your loving-kindness. Without judging yourself, pay attention to how you choose the targets of your loving-kindness.
- Consider that just like you, the person you target has hopes and dreams. They have people in their life whom they love and who love them. Then extend to them wishes for comfort, ease, good health, abundance, and happiness. Try to really feel in your heart the warmth of loving-kindness for this person.
- Notice when loving-kindness shows up naturally, pausing and appreciating it, observing what it feels like in the body. Notice when loving-kindness is more difficult to access.
- It is impossible to do this activity incorrectly. See what your experience is, and let it be what it is. Try this exercise again and again, and notice if extending loving-kindness to strangers gets easier over time. See if you notice any shift in your feeling of connection to others.

CHAPTER 12

Self-Compassion

Though I face challenges
I know I am never alone
I vow to include myself
In the great field of kindness and compassion

In this chapter you will learn how to cultivate compassion for yourself, even in the midst of challenging circumstances. You will be introduced to the "self-compassion break" as an effective intervention for building sustainability in the role of caregiver.

Complete Compassion

In the caregiving courses we teach, a question we often ask caregivers is, "Which is easier, to feel compassion for others or to feel compassion for yourself?" With a few exceptions, participants report that it is easier to direct compassion outward than it is to direct it inward. Which is easier for you?

The meditation teacher Jack Kornfield has said, "If your compassion does not include yourself, it is incomplete." In my observation, the most skillful caregivers are those who use self-compassion as a tool to support themselves through the challenges they face, not just in their caregiver role but in their life generally. Healthy self-compassion supports the caregiver to stay in the care relationship over the long term. Many paid caregivers work in extremely challenging environments. Some family caregivers will provide support to a loved one for many years. It is difficult to imagine how someone can stay in the role of caregiver without a regular self-compassion practice.

I have a dear friend who, like many parents, has faced many challenges caring for her children. I am often in awe of her ability to comfort herself and reset through her self-compassion practice. In fact, I sometimes wonder who she would be without self-compassion. She is fortunate to have learned a very effective practice known as the "self-compassion break," which I will introduce further below. When we talk and she is struggling, she has the lovely ability to name exactly what is happening. She acknowledges that she knows her struggles are common for most parents and that she is trying to be gentle with herself as she recovers from the latest challenge. I can see that this kind of sharing makes her feel a bit lighter, as if she has set down a heavy burden.

As with compassion for others, self-compassion addresses suffering — our own. The experience of self-compassion is similar to the five-stage dynamic process that was described in chapter 9. With self-compassion, it looks only slightly different. As with the first stage of experiencing compassion for others, the first stage of self-compassion is to be aware of suffering. If you do not notice, or want to acknowledge, that you are suffering, you will not embrace self-compassion in helping you with a difficult experience. You will continue to suffer, with the added element of self-delusion or denial. Even if you do not like for others to know you are having difficulties, you can still acknowledge to yourself that you are suffering.

Once you acknowledge to yourself that you are having a tough time, you may have emotional and physical responses to the fact that you are struggling. As discussed in chapter 5, these emotions will manifest in certain parts of your body. The emotions that arise in difficult moments differ from person to person. However, we can say with certainty that everyone experiences some kind of emotional response in difficult situations. Keeping this in mind may help you overcome any shame over what you are going through or any isolation in your experience.

Just as you would want others to be free from suffering, you likely want to alleviate your own suffering. This desire to be free from suffering will motivate you to claim your own agency and do something for yourself. When I experience stress or self-doubt, getting up and moving my body a bit seems to help. However, I need to notice my suffering, and want to do something about it before I can take action to address it. Self-compassion can take the form of self-soothing, or self-coaching. In other words, you give yourself the kind of positive self-talk similar to what you would give to a dear friend who is having a tough time.

Take a moment to imagine a loved one or a friend who is struggling with a particular issue. What would you say to them? How would you express your loving-kindness and support? How would you convey that you want them to be free from suffering? As you imagine yourself expressing your support, notice how it makes you feel in your heart.

Can you imagine soothing or supporting yourself in this same way? Are you any less deserving of your kindness than your loved one or friend? No! However, if it is difficult for you to imagine self-soothing, don't worry. The practice I introduce below will give you what you need.

After directing compassionate action toward yourself, you will likely experience the same warm glow we discussed in chapter 9; however, you may experience it more subtly than if you had directed that compassion outward. Nonetheless, this glow is also important to notice and enjoy. Think of it as a reward for your ability to comfort yourself, so that you can comfort others.

Three Essential Elements of Self-Compassion

The three elements essential to self-compassion are found in the process described above. They are *awareness*, *recognition of common humanity*, and *kindness*. If any of these elements is missing, then you will not fully experience self-compassion.

The self-compassion break is a highly effective practice for meeting a challenge, whether it be feelings of inadequacy, doubt, or overwhelm, making a mistake, saying the wrong thing, dealing with a difficult person, a sense of failure, or anything else that elicits negative thoughts or emotions or causes you to feel stressed. The intervention in this particular form was reimagined by the researcher and professor of educational psychology Kristin Neff, author of *Self Compassion: The Proven Power of Being Kind to Yourself.* The practice has three steps that correspond to the three essential elements of self-compassion.

Before practicing the self-compassion break, it may be helpful to first pause for a moment to imagine yourself in a difficult caregiving situation. It does not need to be the most intense challenge you have faced recently but just something that you have found unsettling. Try to recall what was going on. Who was involved? Where were you? Before you begin the practice, give yourself a moment or two to recall the thoughts and feelings you experienced during the situation.

Awareness

To begin the self-compassion break, take two or three deep intentional breaths. Next, imagining you are back in the situation you just recalled, acknowledge that you are struggling. You might say to yourself, "I am suffering." Or, "Wow! I am having difficulty with this." Or, "I recognize I am struggling here." Find the language that works for you.

This first step is about being completely honest with yourself about what is truly happening. This kind of authenticity is essential to genuine mindful awareness. Neff writes, "Research shows that people with higher levels of self-compassion are more willing to experience their difficult feelings and to acknowledge that their emotions are valid and important." For the self-compassion break to be impactful, you must be willing to see, accept, and experience the truth of your circumstances and your emotional response. When you have an effective way of dealing with negative emotions, you will not resist them or pretend you are not having them. By acknowledging your true emotional experience, you strengthen your ability to let whatever emotions arise play out naturally.

Common Humanity

Following your acknowledgment of suffering, remind yourself that to be human means that you will inevitably encounter difficulty. Remind yourself that everyone suffers in one way or another. And, although the details of your circumstances may be unique, you are not alone in the experience of suffering. Silently say to yourself, "Everyone struggles from time to time. I am not alone." Or, "Caregiving is not easy. Like other caregivers, I too struggle." Find the phrase that is right for you in acknowledging your shared humanity, not only with other caregivers but with all human beings. At this point you might pause and think of all the caregivers in the world who also face hardships in their role.

Kindness

Finally, after acknowledging your suffering and your shared humanity, offer kindness to yourself. If it is comfortable for you, place a hand, or both hands, on your chest over your heart. Notice the sensations of this contact. Say to yourself, "May I be kind to myself in this experience of suffering." Or, "As I struggle, may I hold my experience with kindness." It could be, "With kindness, I've got this." Whatever phrase feels authentic to you.

You might pause at this final stage of the self-compassion break and ask yourself, "What act of kindness toward myself would be most nurturing?" Consider what your aching heart, your exhausted body, or your agitated mind needs at this moment. Depending on your caregiving situation, your options may be limited. If you are constrained in any way by your circumstances, find what is possible. Although you might benefit most from a warm bath, a nap, or a long vacation, you can also try to find more accessible and immediate expressions of kindness toward yourself. Even the simple phrase "I've got this" will support you to carry on and reclaim your agency, your confidence, and your self-worth. No matter what form it takes, self-compassion builds your capacity to meet whatever struggles you encounter.

The self-compassion break is highly effective for moving through any challenge with honesty and strength. It is a mental and emotional reset. What I love about this practice is that it is discreet; you can do it without anyone around you even noticing. The more you use the self-compassion break, the more natural it becomes. Eventually, you won't even have to remember to apply self-compassion; it will be automatic. The self-compassion break will become part of your toolkit for thriving in the role of caregiver. With self-compassion, you become your best advocate.

Blocked Self-Compassion

For some caregivers, cultivating self-compassion will feel impossible. Maybe you have been told that you are not worthy of compassion, and you are convinced this is true. Or perhaps you believe you have hurt others and so you deserve punishment in the form of denying yourself compassion. You may have a deeply held belief that self-compassion is weak or indulgent. Overcoming these beliefs may be challenging and will take time. But it is more than worth it.

If you find it difficult to generate self-compassion, try acknowledging the truth of this blockage. Then acknowledge that such difficulty is also true for others. Finally, see if you can let go of any judgment about your inability to direct compassion toward yourself. Take your time with the self-compassion practice. Consider taking one step at a time over the course of several days. If you can't get there, keep moving through the book, but tag this chapter and come back to it when you are ready to try again.

One technique that may work if you find it challenging to direct compassion to yourself is to visualize yourself as a small child. You might even keep an old photo of yourself with you until the practice of self-compassion becomes more familiar and automatic. That innocent and vulnerable child you visualize or see in the photo is still there within you. Every child is worthy of compassion. Direct your compassion toward that little one inside.

Another way to work with a blockage toward self-compassion is to fake it. That is, go through the steps of the self-compassion break, even if the feelings of warmth are not there, and see what happens. It will not harm you! You may start to notice that the practice helps you feel better about yourself, especially in challenging situations.

The relationship between self-compassion and compassion toward others is another reflection of the reciprocity of caregiving covered in chapter 10. Building the capacity to be with suffering begins with your own. When you tend to your own needs, you can show up more fully for others. You learn a lot about comforting others by learning how to soothe yourself. As the old teacher told the young monk, "Serve others by serving yourself."

I am sure the person you are caring for, if asked, would say they want you to attend to your own emotional and physical needs. Given that they are likely quite dependent on you, it makes sense that they would want you to be you well-resourced with tools and practices that sustain you in your role as caregiver. Someday you may need to depend on the support of a caregiver. Will you want the support of a caregiver who is unable to maintain their own well-being?

We all benefit from practicing self-compassion. Denying the need for self-compassion is like disconnecting the fuel gauge on your car. You can pretend you won't run out of gas; however, sooner or later you will run out of fuel, and when you do, you will have to deal with the problems it causes for both you and your passengers.

[Practice]

Begin to work with the self-compassion break whenever you encounter an internal or external difficulty. Find the phrase for each of the three steps that works best for you. Notice how you feel after applying self-compassion when encountering a challenging situation.

The three steps of the self-compassion break:

1. **Awareness:** "I am suffering." Think about how you are suffering.

2. **Common humanity:** "Everyone struggles from time to time. I am not alone." Think of the endless numbers of caregivers who, just like you, face difficulties.
3. **Kindness:** "In this experience of suffering, may I be kind to myself." Place one or both hands on your chest over your heart. Consider what small gesture of kindness toward yourself would be supportive.

CHAPTER 13

Barriers to Compassion

I am a compassionate caregiver
Yet I know obstacles will get in my way
May I honor the truth of what shows up
And find the way back to my most authentic self

[**Blocked compassion is extremely common. Barriers to compassion show up for a variety of reasons, which will be identified and explained in this chapter.**]

I was talking with Hana shortly after her father was transferred from his home to our residential hospice house. As we sat together away from her father's room, she explained that she was very relieved to finally have him in a place where she no longer had to take care of him. Hana shared that she didn't think she would visit very much. I learned that her father had always been very demanding and mean-spirited. After her mother died, Hana was thrown into caring for him. Although she was very angry with her father over how he treated both her and her mother, Hana felt responsible for looking after him.

Now that her father was in a place where others could look after his needs, Hana was finished with him. She said she could no longer force herself to be around him. Despite saying she was relieved, I could clearly see Hana was distressed. I believe she wanted to be compassionate toward her father, but too much resentment and anger were getting in the way. I assured Hana that her father was in good hands and encouraged her to take care of herself.

This story is not unusual. It is quite common for our compassion to become blocked by some internal barrier. Human relationships are extremely complex, and it can sometimes be difficult to rise above past or present difficulties to become kind and compassionate. Blocked compassion does not mean you are a bad person or lacking in compassion. You are only human. Thankfully, barriers to compassion can usually be overcome.

As you read in chapter 9, the five-part dynamic process of compassion begins with the awareness of suffering. It is also the case that overcoming a barrier to compassion begins with being aware of the barrier. Once you are aware of the emotion, attitude, or physical sensation interfering with your compassion, you can begin to work with it. I have noticed for myself that bringing awareness to the barrier will often allow me to move beyond it. This chapter looks at various barriers and how they disrupt compassion in the context of caregiving. The next chapter will address ways to overcome barriers and what to do when overcoming them is not possible. For now, just notice if any of the barriers described below seem familiar to you in your role of caregiver.

Perfectionism

If you are a caregiver who will do something perfectly or not at all, your compassion may get blocked when you see suffering that you believe requires action beyond your skills. Or maybe you only have so much time and you think that to adequately address the suffering you see, more time is needed than what you have. So you let things be and do nothing.

Once when I was visiting with my friend Marilyn, she expressed sadness over no longer being able to do social justice work like she used to. Her inability to get involved in issues important to her contributed to her belief that she had no purpose in life. I mentioned a campaign to send out postcards to encourage people to vote and to become engaged in local issues. Marilyn perked up and asked what organization was sponsoring the campaign. Although she could no longer do many of the things she once enjoyed, Marilyn was certainly capable of writing postcards from her home. I told her I would send her some information. Following our visit, a couple busy days went by as I waited to find the free time to thoroughly research organizations sponsoring this kind of volunteer work. I wanted to send her a list of campaigns to choose from. Finally, I told myself there will never be a good time to do this amount of research, so I went online and found two organizations and sent an email off to Marilyn. It was not perfect, but two organizations had to be enough. When I saw her afterward, she expressed her appreciation that I had sent her at least some information.

Judgment

Although judgment can be subtle, it is still very disruptive to compassion. You may find that judgment arises when you think about what caused the circumstances the person you care for is dealing with. Or you may judge their habits that in your opinion make their situation worse. An attitude of "why should I do anything for them if they aren't going to do anything for themself" may arise for you.

Rooted in judgment is the experience of "empathic collapse." Empathic collapse occurs when you view the person who is suffering as different from you, and thus you do not experience the kind of empathy you would for someone you perceive to be the same as you. There is a rich body of research on this type of "othering" and how it impacts compassion. Psychologist and researcher Susan Fiske developed a social cognition model that offers insight into why we categorize others in ways that influence our behavior toward them, including whether we can act with compassion. She shows that we treat people differently depending on the subtle biases we hold about them. Without going into detail here about social cognition, I simply encourage you to notice when and if you lack empathy because you judge someone to be different from you.

Compassion Fatigue

You have likely heard the term *compassion fatigue* before, especially in the context of healthcare. The Covid pandemic brought this issue front and center. We have heard countless stories of healthcare workers feeling overwhelmed by the scale of suffering they encountered at their hospitals. Many caregivers left their jobs because of this overwhelm.

Compassion fatigue entails no longer feeling good about the impact you may be having because the scale of suffering you confront is so great. You assume you can't possibly make a difference when so much suffering is taking place around you. Or you assume that no matter how much you give, it will never be enough. Someone experiencing compassion fatigue loses sight of the impact of small acts, so they stop acting to alleviate suffering. While physical exhaustion may contribute to compassion fatigue, it is mostly centered in the thinking mind and can lead to caregiver burnout.

Guilt

Witnessing the struggles of the person you are caring for may cause you to reflect on the history of your relationship. Such reflection may trigger guilt or remorse over past behavior, including not doing more when you had the chance. And these feelings can get in the way of compassion. You may turn away from the suffering so as not to be reminded of past behavior.

Thoughts of the future can also contribute to a guilt-related blockage. You may worry that your compassionate action will be perceived by others as too little too late or as hypocritical. To avoid the judgment of those who may be aware of your past behavior, you do not take compassionate action. You may worry that you will get called out, even though it is never too late to express compassion. It is always a noble and righteous act.

Another situation in which guilt may get in the way of compassionate action is when you see suffering you think requires more than you can provide. Feeling guilty that you cannot do what you think is needed, you do nothing. Perhaps you feel guilt for not being strong enough, for not having the resources, or for lacking the expertise you think is required, so you do nothing.

Embarrassment

Some caregivers may feel embarrassed when they know strangers will witness certain acts of compassion, so to avoid drawing attention to themselves, they don't take actions that might be visible to others. They may want to avoid a "scene" or a misunderstanding. Offering assistance to a stranger who appears to be mentally or emotionally unstable can be a vulnerable or awkward experience, as the usual social rules of engagement may not apply. Or you might hesitate to offer aid to an injured person due to fear of being judged for not knowing how to help. Wanting to protect the image you project into the world is understandable and common. Our egos are powerful checks on our behavior. This concern over what others may notice takes us out of present-moment awareness, where compassion flourishes.

Resentment/Anger

The story at the beginning of this chapter of Hana, the woman angry with her father, is a perfect example of how anger can get in the way of acting compassionately. You may feel she was justified in her decision to leave the care of her father to others, but remember, compassion flourishes in present-moment awareness. Her anger was rooted in her father's past behavior. That does not mean she was being unreasonable. I could see she needed respite from being his caregiver. Yet had she been able to stay focused on the present moment, she may have been able to continue visiting him. Staying in present-moment awareness is especially difficult with someone who has caused us pain in the past.

Familial relationships are rarely simple or straightforward. Resentment toward a parent, sibling, or even a child can be persistent. You may harbor resentment for how you have been treated by the family member you are caring for, and their suffering may feel like some form of justice. Withholding your compassionate action when it could alleviate suffering may feel like a form of payback for past transgressions. Pointing out this kind of barrier to compassion is not to suggest that your anger is not valid; rather, it is to help bring awareness of what is truly happening if you experience this. You cannot overcome a barrier if you are not aware of it.

You compassion can get blocked even when you are on the receiving end of anger. You may hesitate to act compassionately toward the person who is angry with you, thinking the offer of assistance will worsen, or reignite, their anger.

Fear

You may find that your compassion gets blocked when you fear that what you do to address the suffering may worsen the situation for the one who suffers. You may fear that you will make a mistake and somehow harm the person you are trying to support. Or you may be fearful of harming yourself in the process of acting compassionately.

In such situations, it may not be readily clear how to best proceed with compassion. I recall instances when a resident at the guest house facility wanted to go outside. It was possible that this would be their last opportunity to be outdoors. When I first began volunteering there, the two-story house did not have an elevator. Getting some residents up or down meant two or more caregivers had to carry someone in a wheelchair down the long staircase. There were times when I had to weigh taking a chance on honoring their wish to get downstairs against disappointing them but keeping them safe upstairs.

The barrier of fear is not always a negative thing. Sometimes it serves a useful purpose. Having your compassion disrupted by fear may result in your taking a less desirable course of action. However, what at first glance seems like a less desirable course of action may actually be the most appropriate act of compassion. Compassion does not mean you always proceed in the way the person suffering wants you to. Their disappointment or displeasure does not mean you did not act compassionately.

Another common fear that can block compassionate action is when you believe taking measures to alleviate suffering will trigger a cascade of events that changes life significantly for you and the person you care for. And the fear causes you to avoid acknowledging the seriousness of the suffering you witness. Examples of this type of fear blockage may be avoiding the decision to initiate your loved one's move into an assisted-living facility or putting off scheduling a doctor's appointment to look into a concerning new issue your loved one is dealing with. Being blocked by either the barrier of fear or the barrier of anticipatory grief (addressed below) can look a lot like denial.

I will never forget the morning my father called to express concern about my mother. As I drove toward work, my dad explained to me that my mom was slurring her words. I asked him to pass the phone to her. Although she was understandable, I noticed that her speech was indeed slurred. She did not seem distressed, and that in itself was very worrisome. It was as if she could not see that anything was wrong. My mother and I spoke for a few minutes before I asked her to put my dad back on the line.

Although I did not want to alarm my father, I conveyed to him as calmly as possible that I thought he needed to call an ambulance. He paused for a moment before replying that he was going to wait a while to see how things went. I pushed back. I don't think he wanted to say out loud that he was negotiating with my mom. Closing our conversation, he told me he would call the ambulance.

I don't judge my father for the way he handled that situation with my mother. I was in California, and they were in the Detroit area in the house I grew up in. I can't judge him when I was so far removed from their day-to-day realities. It was not until several hours later, after other conversations with me and my siblings, that my dad called for an ambulance.

Mom went right into the emergency department and from there

into the hospital's intensive care unit. That night, I was on a plane to Detroit. The strange conversation I had with my mom as I was driving into work was the last one I had with her. Looking back on that day, I think my father was fearful of what this new development would bring to their lives, so he avoided the compassionate action that was called for. It is easy to imagine that he was also fearful of upsetting my mother. I know in my heart that on that morning, my dad wanted to do the right thing to lessen my mom's suffering; however, it took him time to bring himself to move from intention to action. We later learned that my mother was experiencing congestive heart failure, which caused cerebral hypoxia, or insufficient oxygen flow to the brain, causing the slurred speech.

Avoidance of Anticipatory Grief

Being a caregiver means you bear witness to the progression of illness. You see the subtle changes the person you are caring for goes through over an extended period of time. Certain episodes of suffering may bring the trajectory of their prognosis into clear focus, and this may cause anticipatory grief, or grief that begins before a loved one dies. Perhaps you begin to see the ways both your life and the life of the person you care for will change; some plans may no longer be realistic, certain freedoms are lost, or pieces of long-held identity break down. You may begin grieving not just the loss of the person you care for but also the ways life is changing.

When a loved one has a serious illness, anticipatory grief can hide just under the surface. Then an acute episode of suffering can bring that grief to the surface. As you likely have experienced yourself, grief is often difficult and messy. Profound grief tends to influence every aspect of life, and this is why so many people try to pretend it is not arising or attempt to push it off to later. If you try to avoid anticipatory grief by denying the suffering you witness, you will not respond to the situation with compassionate action.

Revulsion or Disgust

While I was serving on the hospice ward at the city hospital, a man named Jim lived in the ward. Jim had a large cancerous tumor on one side of his face. Over time, his condition worsened and the tumor grew. Of course, the side of Jim's face was kept dressed in bandages. I rarely saw anyone other than the nurses spend time with him, unlike most of the residents.

Jim reached a point when areas of the tumor cells began dying, causing a horrible odor. His suffering was very obvious to everyone. And seeing his suffering caused me emotional distress. Looking back on the situation, I realize the only thing I could have done to alleviate his suffering was to spend time with him. That was the compassionate action I could have taken. Although I wanted to see his suffering decreased, I could not bring myself to approach him. Regretfully, I was simply too put off by the horrible smell.

Each caregiver will respond differently to conditions like foul odors, unpleasant-looking wounds, or disabilities. Even strange sounds like gurgling or moaning can be off-putting. It can be difficult to overcome emotional or physical reactions to things we find disgusting. And when we react negatively to unpleasant sights, sounds, and smells, our best intentions to act compassionately may be blocked.

Exhaustion

You have very likely discovered for yourself that caregiving can be exhausting. Even young and healthy caregivers have days of not feeling quite up for what is expected of them. When you are overly exhausted due to lack of sleep, working long hours, or illness, you will not be very inclined to offer compassionate action to address the suffering experienced by the person you are caring for. You may feel taking compassionate action will ask too much of you. It is natural to be protective of yourself when you are tired. You may consciously or subconsciously conserve your energy and withdraw inward a bit. When you are tired, you may expect the person you care to do much more for themselves.

As we know, a contributing factor to caregiver exhaustion is inadequate self-care. If you notice that your compassion is getting blocked due to exhaustion, you may want to look at your relationship to self-care. Maintaining healthy self-care practices is extremely difficult for many caregivers, since often their responsibilities do not leave much time to focus on this.

Despite how difficult it can be for caregivers to make time for adequate self-care, it needs to be acknowledged that poor self-care will catch up with them sooner or later. Failing to tend to your own emotional and physical health affects not only your well-being but also that of the person benefiting from your care. We will look more closely at self-care in the final section of the book, where you will find some ideas for integrating self-care into a busy schedule.

Moral Distress

The barrier of moral distress is primarily relevant to paid caregivers working in a facility or a hospital system or doing in-home care. Moral distress is ultimately the result of external or systemic factors that interfere with a caregiver's desire to address the suffering they witness. The caregiver may be inclined to act with compassion, but workplace conditions make it impossible. Under these circumstances, the caregiver may want to give up. It may be easier for them to look away from suffering than to oppose or make peace with the conditions or policies dictating their care.

One example of a situation that might contribute to moral distress is the requirement to maintain a high caseload of patients, preventing a caregiver from spending enough time comforting a grieving patient or family member. Another is when a paid caregiver is told by a family member not to do something for a patient that the caregiver knows would benefit them, such as taking the patient for a longer walk than the family member believes is appropriate. Or perhaps a caregiver may believe that the person they are caring for would benefit from a particular medical device but discover that the device is not covered by insurance and too costly to purchase.

Empathic Distress

In chapter 9 we looked at the five-stage process of experiencing compassion, and we differentiated between empathy and compassion. I mentioned that some caregivers get stuck at the second, empathic, stage of compassion and do not progress further. In order to move from empathy to compassionate action, you must be able to differentiate between the suffering you witness and your own emotional experience. In other words, if you take on others' suffering, making it your own, you may not feel motivated to take action to alleviate the suffering. If you find that your empathy leads to distress, you are probably focused on protecting yourself from uncomfortable emotions and not on the ways you might alleviate the suffering you witness.

Those who study the relationship between empathy and compassion find that often what is labeled compassion fatigue is actually empathic distress. I do not think it is possible to exhaust your compassion; however, a constant state of empathic distress from taking on the suffering of others can lead you to believe that your compassion is depleted.

The psychology and neuroscience researchers Tania Singer and Olga Klimecki explain that "while empathy refers to our general capacity to resonate with others' emotional states...empathic distress refers to a strong aversive and self-oriented response to the suffering of others, accompanied by the desire to withdraw from a situation in order to protect oneself from excessive feelings." When you become aware of suffering and you have an empathic response, you have two possible paths. The first path is being oriented to others, which leads to compassionate action, and the second is being self-oriented, which leads to negative emotions and distress. The second path is essentially getting stuck in empathy without the outlet of compassionate action.

Emotional Hijack

In some situations, such as emergencies, you may find that your compassionate action is blocked by a temporary flood of strong emotions.

Daniel Goleman, psychologist and author of *Emotional Intelligence: Why It Can Matter More Than IQ*, labels such episodes as "amygdala hijacks." The amygdala is part of the brain's limbic system, the part of the brain involved in emotional and behavioral responses to external stimuli. Your brain may respond to certain events automatically before you have a chance to think through the best response to them. The automatic response of the amygdala overpowers, or hijacks, your rational thinking.

My sister recently shared a story about her mother-in-law, who was dealing with a serious illness and fainted. My sister, who is typically a take-charge kind of person, completely froze. She was temporarily unable to think through what to do next. Thankfully, her husband was present and was able to address his mother's needs. Freezing is one of three primary acute stress responses. The others, fight or flight, are most likely familiar to you.

In the context of caregiving, freezing is the most common acute stress response you will encounter. This is a state of momentary panic. When the amygdala hijacks your brain, it is overriding the frontal cortex part of the brain that processes rational thinking. In these intense situations it is common to lose the ability to think straight or access working memory.

Only (Super) Human

I view caregivers as superhuman in that they perform absolutely incredible feats in caring for others. It is also true that caregivers are only human and are thus imperfect. Even if you have experienced every one of the barriers mentioned above, do not be discouraged. Over time, it will become easier for you to identify the barrier blocking your compassion and to take steps to overcome it. Most important in overcoming compassion barriers is being aware of what is happening when you are blocked. Always start with awareness.

Overcoming barriers to compassion comes with a substantial payoff. More and more research shows that by deepening your compassion, you increase purpose and happiness in your role as a caregiver and in life generally. People who act to address the needs of others also enjoy many physical health benefits, such as lower blood pressure, lower levels of inflammation, increased cardiovascular health, and even longer life. In the next chapter, I will share ways to overcome the barriers that get in the way of acting compassionately toward others.

[Practice]

Take a moment to reflect on your relationship with the person you care for. Ask yourself if your compassion toward this person has recently been blocked. Try to identify the barriers that have gotten in the way of extending compassion. Write down the particular barriers that have shown up for you. Are there one or two barriers that arise more often than others?

Be on the lookout for moments when your compassion toward others becomes blocked. Reflect on what is getting in the way. If you are unable to move past the barrier obstructing your compassion, notice if self-judgment arises, and if so, try to shift into self-compassion.

CHAPTER 14

Overcoming Barriers to Compassion

Returning to compassion
I find my true home
Finding joy and meaning
In my essential connection to all beings

Noticing that your compassion is blocked also means you are noticing the suffering of the person you are caring for. However, you still may not be able to move from awareness of suffering to action because your thoughts about that action are disrupting your instinct to do something. An unsettled mind makes it very difficult to act with compassion. In this chapter you will discover how to overcome the barriers named in the last chapter.

When thoughts are negative or simply distracting, they disrupt the heart's natural inclination to address others' needs with kindness and compassion. In Buddhist teachings, the unruly mind is often compared to demons wreaking havoc on one's peace of mind and sense of true self. I can relate to this comparison. When negative or even just unhelpful thoughts persist, it feels as though I am in battle against dark forces taking over my thoughts and sensations. It takes a lot of effort to quiet a busy mind, especially when someone we care for is suffering and action is needed. To overcome any barriers to compassion, it is helpful to step back and observe our thoughts.

In many Asian cultures, the word *mind* is associated not only with the thinking mind or the brain but also with the heart. In those cultures, head and heart are inseparable. However you view this relationship, is it clear that our thoughts influence whether or not we can respond from the heart.

Since most of the barriers to compassion are rooted in thoughts, managing the influence of thoughts on your capacity for compassion requires that you master metacognition. This is the state of awareness we first covered in chapter 3 when we discussed stepping back and becoming the observer of your thoughts and feelings. When you notice that your compassion is blocked, take a moment to notice what is happening in your thinking mind. Ask yourself, "What thoughts are interfering with my compassion? Are the thoughts protecting my physical well-being or my ego? Are the thoughts factual in this moment?"

Once you have accomplished the important first step of simply observing the thoughts blocking your compassion, how you respond to these last two questions will offer you a path forward. If you determine that your thoughts are really about protecting your ego and not your physical well-being, it may be easier to let the thoughts go and take action. Or if you can be honest with yourself and see that your thoughts do not represent objective reality, you may be able to push past them and extend an act of compassion that addresses the needs of the moment.

If you determine that your thoughts are actually about protecting your physical well-being, your compassionate action will look different than if your thoughts are about protecting your ego or emotional state. Consider the story shared in the previous chapter about the very real risk of getting weak patients up and down the stairs. Even though you may not be able to do what you believe is needed out of fear for your safety or that of the one you are caring for, there are still actions you can take.

Let's consider some ways to overcome the barriers mentioned in the last chapter.

Perfectionism, Judgment, and Compassion Fatigue

We will look at perfectionism, judgment, and compassion fatigue together, since they are each primarily thought experiences, with a secondary emotional and/or physical component.

When you notice your compassion is blocked and realize your thoughts are focused on attaining perfection, judging the one who is suffering, or not making a difference no matter what you do, it is time to disrupt these thoughts by shifting your focus from thinking mind to sensing mind. By focusing on your sensations, you come back to what is true in the moment. Although your thoughts are important and feel very real to you, they are not necessarily an accurate reflection of reality. Your thoughts are shaped by many filters informed by a lifetime of experiences and conditioning. In my experience, what I think is true about a particular situation or interaction often proves to be inaccurate.

Turning your attention to the direct experience of sensations, you shift into present-moment awareness. You can ask yourself, "What do I feel in my body?" "What sounds do I hear in my environment?" "What do I see or smell?" "What do I feel on my skin?" Compassion thrives in present-moment awareness where arising experience is complete and perfect just as it is, and there is no room for judgment or doubt. If you can let go of thoughts that seek perfection, cast judgment, or make you doubt your impact, your unfiltered heart will guide you back to doing something to alleviate suffering. When you act from a place of love, you don't worry about being perfect, you don't need to feel special by judging others as different from you, and you don't doubt the impact of your actions, understanding that our world is desperate for any act of compassion, no matter how insignificant it may seem.

Guilt, Embarrassment, Resentment/Anger, and Fear

I consider guilt, embarrassment, resentment/anger, and fear similar emotions in the context of caregiving since they are all informed by our thoughts. Reflecting on what has happened or what may happen triggers these emotional barriers to compassion. With each of these barriers, thoughts get in the way of taking the action that is an essential part of genuine compassion. You may still notice suffering and even have an empathic response; however, negative emotions will interfere with your ability to carry out all the stages of compassion.

Overcoming any of these barriers requires the approaches we covered in chapter 5, where we looked at managing big emotions. Disrupting the thoughts that trigger blocking emotions allows you to drop into a state of being where the mind is settled and you are motivated by a clear and open heart. In *A Fearless Heart*, Thupten Jinpa emphasizes the importance of cultivating a quiet attentive mind in order to be more available for the care of others:

> We learn to unhook our awareness from the restless, tiresome activity of habitual thought patterns and from our instinctive and automatic emotional reactions to these. We learn to quiet the ceaseless internal chatter of what-ifs, and we learn to let go of the over-interpreting, ruminating, and clinging to our experiences.... A quiet(er) mind is a place we can more readily be present, which makes us available to care for ourselves and others.

Once you step back and notice that you are experiencing one of these big emotions, you are already in a place of awareness. You know that your emotions are disrupting your compassion. Now you can drop into a state of present-moment awareness and begin quieting the mind. See if doing so shifts your motivation to take compassionate action. If the emotions persist, return to physical sensations to quiet the mind again. Keep coming back to the place of open mind and open heart.

When one of these emotions blocks your compassion, it may be helpful to ask yourself what you would need if the roles were reversed. If your caregiver was experiencing the same emotion as you, what would you hope to see from them? Would you want them to rise above it all and act to alleviate your suffering? Keep in mind that in the case of guilt or resentment, acting compassionately does not require you to first forgive yourself or the person you are caring for. Forgiveness is not a prerequisite to acting with compassion. However, offering compassion to someone you have hurt or to someone who has hurt you may make forgiveness easier to access.

In the case of embarrassment, it may be helpful to think about past experiences of witnessing someone in public extending compassion to another in need. How did it make you feel? Did any negative judgment arise for you? Probably not. For much of my life, I have avoided situations that could cause me embarrassment. Then I began to realize that I was not all that important to strangers. Basically, I got over myself. Avoiding embarrassment, or someone's harsh judgment, is very much about protecting your ego. Your ego may get harmed in embarrassing situations, and while the temporary emotional pain of a bruised ego is real, it is certainly different from physical harm. We can more easily overcome a bruised ego when we experience the warm glow that follows an act of compassion.

Anticipatory Grief

When your compassion gets blocked by avoiding anticipatory grief, you are likely resisting action that may remind you of what might happen in the future. No one wants to experience grief, whether it is anticipatory or due to a loss that has already occurred. Part of the reason many of us so fiercely avoid grief is that we have not developed the capacity to cope with big emotional experiences. While learning emotional skills is vital to providing good care and to being happy, it is also true that some grief is so profound and painful that no amount of preparation or skill will make things easier. We will look at profound and complicated grief a bit later in the book.

Overcoming the barrier of avoiding anticipatory grief is also about shifting attention away from troubling thoughts and coming back to present-moment awareness by attuning to sensations. Anticipatory grief is activated by thoughts, in particular, thoughts that project you into the future. If you can focus on what is true in the moment, you should be able to move through this barrier and extend compassion. Redirecting your attention is not about denying the emotions that arise for you when you think about your future loss but about turning back to the fullness of what is still here. Your loved one may be suffering greatly, and because you are human, you know where all this is heading; however, you are also capable of recognizing that what is here, no matter what it looks like, is worthy of your gratitude and attention. Let your compassionate action express your love for what is still here, knowing that it too, like everything, will be taken.

It may also be helpful to remind yourself that you will have plenty of time to work with your grief later, but for now, your thoughts and actions should be about living as fully as possible. When you look back on your experience of caring for a loved one, will you regret not spending more time grieving before they died? Or will you regret that you did not have more opportunities to express your love? Let your love propel you into taking compassionate action now.

Revulsion/Disgust and Exhaustion

If you are a direct-care worker or a clinician, you know that over time you become used to being around the unpleasant conditions and symptoms that can be part of caring for someone living with illness. For some caregivers, turning away from things they find disgusting is just not an option. Showing up for such situations is a requirement of employment. Or a family caregiver may not have anyone else to call on who can deal with a situation that requires immediate attention.

One approach I have found useful is to remind myself that I am here to serve and that the needs of the person suffering are my priority. In other words, it is not about me. Another expression of compassion is doing whatever possible to maintain the dignity of the person who is suffering. This is not to suggest that you should push past your limits, as that can also be harmful. However, reframing a situation to prioritize the dignity of the person you care for may be what is needed to overcome the resistance you experience when witnessing something that causes disgust.

It can also be helpful to acknowledge to the person you are caring for that you are having a tough time with what you find unpleasant or disgusting. If you can do it skillfully, naming out loud how you are feeling to the person needing your compassionate attention can help you push through resistance. You might say something like, "I am so sorry you are dealing with this situation. I am finding it a bit difficult to support you right now, but I am committed to being here. Please forgive me if I need to approach this slowly." I have cared for people who had no control over their bowels, and the smell was overwhelming. It always seemed to me that the person suffering appreciated my honesty. Once I had named out loud what was true, we were both able to move beyond the awkwardness and just be with the experience. There is power in acknowledging the truth of what is rather than denying or avoiding it.

On a more practical level, I have learned some tricks from nurses to help decrease the severity of a disgust reaction. Some nurses use a small amount of Vicks VapoRub under their nose to block a bad odor, or they spray a lot of room freshener. Breathing through your mouth can also help. Sometimes just taking practical steps can unblock a compassion barrier.

Always remember that you are only human, and the emotion of disgust is very common. It is a basic human emotion that has helped us survive by guiding us to avoid things that are harmful. Being kind to yourself will make it easier for you to accept whatever may be triggering your disgust.

Like disgust, exhaustion primarily has a physical component. When you are exhausted, it is natural to self-protect by seeking rest or avoiding exertion. When you simply cannot give any more due to exhaustion, practice self-compassion. Finding a way to rest and rejuvenate is an act of compassion that supports not only you but also the person you care for. Your exhaustion is not doing them any good.

Also, as mentioned earlier, focusing your attention and energy on what is in front of you when you are tired may allow you to stay with your caregiving until you are able to rest. Remember, a busy mind contributes to exhaustion. When you are so exhausted that you cannot go on, it helps to accept that while you rest, things may take place that are beyond your control. You cannot be responsible for everything all the time, and to think otherwise is unrealistic. Like anyone else, you have your limits. Hopefully you can find solace in knowing that you are doing what you can, and that more is just not possible.

Moral Distress

Moral distress is caused by externally imposed barriers, so there may not be much you can do to change your circumstances. This does not mean you cannot act compassionately to address suffering, just not all the suffering you see. You will be able to attend to some experiences of suffering and not others. So it becomes essential to focus on the worthiness of the compassion you are able to extend rather than on what you are unable to do. Remember that even small acts of compassion can improve things for someone who is suffering. If you cannot spend time with someone you believe would benefit from your companionship, can you at least greet them with warmheartedness? I know that when I am struggling, even a friendly smile from a kind stranger feels really wonderful.

Empathic Distress

Many years ago, I met Lin Maslow, an extremely skillful nurse who also happened to be a Zen priest. At the time, Lin was working as a hospice nurse. I learned a lot from him about integrating mindfulness and compassion into caring for others. One thing that stands out to me is an idea he referred to as "compassionate detachment." This concept reminds us that although we are all connected, and when others suffer we suffer too, it is also true that becoming enmeshed in another's suffering will block or complicate our compassionate response. Lin shared, "Compassionate detachment means we recognize that we are not responsible for the causes and conditions of another person's suffering." In other words, although you may be impacted when you witness another's suffering, you need to recognize it is not *your* suffering. But this kind of compassionate detachment is not a reason to withhold compassion.

If you have trouble discerning the difference between the suffering you witness and your own suffering, you will experience empathic distress. When you are caring for a close family member or a dear friend, it is natural to have an emotional response to their suffering. This only becomes a problem when you are swept up in your own emotional pain and a resulting desire to protect yourself instead of shifting into other-orientation and addressing the suffering you witness.

Every now and then I hear from caregivers that they do not want to join a class or support group because they can't bear to hear about the struggles of other caregivers. They feel they are too overwhelmed by their own challenges to hear about the challenges faced by others. This is an example of how empathic distress blocks compassion. If these caregivers were to find a way to shift out of avoidance and into supportive action that entails being present and listening, they would likely experience positive emotions that combat the negative impacts of stressful or difficult caregiving.

Part of the reason caregivers experience empathic distress is that they have not developed the skills enabling them to experience present-moment awareness and to manage difficult emotions. As discussed in chapter 5, as soon as you notice that you are having negative emotions in response to another's suffering, you can choose to disrupt the thoughts that are triggering the emotions by shifting your attention to physical sensations. Once you stabilize your mind and your emotions, you should be able to shift into other-orientation and find a way to alleviate suffering.

Emotional Hijack

A sudden overwhelming flood of emotions may temporarily block your ability to take action in an emergency. However, there are things you can do in such situations to shorten the duration of a hijack. Applying mindfulness will support you in these kinds of situations. The STOP practice you learned in chapter 8 is a perfect intervention for shortening the duration of a freeze response:

- **Stop.**
- **Take a breath,** or two or three.
- **Observe** physical sensations. A moment or two of keeping your attention on the body should be long enough to regulate your emotions.
- **Proceed** once you regain a state of calm awareness. You should now be able to take action.

The more you practice cultivating mindful awareness, the easier it will be to prevent hijacks and to regulate your emotions when you experience a hijacking.

Self-Compassion in Overcoming Barriers

In chapter 13 I offered some ways to overcome resistance to extending compassion to yourself. In this chapter we will look at the role self-compassion plays in dealing with the barriers mentioned above.

When you notice your compassion being blocked, do your best to be easy on yourself. Try to minimize the time you spend in self-judging thoughts. Remember that you are only human, and thus you are fallible. You have shortcomings just like the rest of us. When outward-facing compassion is blocked, expressing compassion toward yourself may be just what is needed for you to push through the barrier. You may need to remind yourself that it is okay to tend to your own needs before you can tend to those of others.

Recognizing that your compassion is blocked may cause you distress. If it does, simply acknowledge that it does, and take a moment to engage in the three steps of the self-compassion break. Silently or out loud, acknowledge to yourself that you are having a difficult time, remember that others also experience barriers to compassion, and finally, express kindness to yourself. If the self-compassion break does not allow you to move through the barrier, continue expressing compassion to yourself. Try to stay open to the possibility that something will shift.

Giving and Receiving

Sometimes we underestimate the power of pure presence in alleviating suffering. There may be times when you just do not know what to do to alleviate the suffering of the person you are caring for. Or perhaps the person you care for is nearing death, and there is nothing more you can do. In these situations, an impactful and compassionate act may be to engage in a practice that is known as *tonglen*, or "giving and receiving."

Giving and receiving practice is a wonderful way to express both compassion and loving-kindness. It affirms our recognition that although we do not need to make someone else's suffering our own, we are also not separate from it. Giving and receiving puts us in direct relationship to those we care for while opening the heart. I have been in situations when the suffering I am witnessing has felt like too much for me. Perhaps the person I am with is in extreme pain or expressing intense grief, or they are conveying a story of horrible abuse. In those moments my mind can get busy figuring out how I can get away from the suffering before me. In those moments, applying the giving and receiving practice has allowed me to settle my mind and continue bearing witness for one more breath.

In giving and receiving, you begin by resting your attention on your breath for a moment or two. Then, when you feel settled, with the exhale silently extend your wishes for comfort, ease, and happiness to the person you are with. It may be helpful to imagine these wishes carried within a warm bright light released from your heart. Then, on the inhale, receive from them all the suffering they are experiencing. You may want to imagine their suffering as dark clouds, if that feels safe for you. Let your mind and body transform struggles into ease as you inhale suffering and exhale kindness. If at any point you begin to feel overwhelmed by the suffering you receive, remember that a courageous, open heart is always more powerful than suffering. I find it helpful to think about how on cold days my body transforms the cold air I inhale into the warm air I exhale. Let your heart transform suffering into ease. If breathing in the dark cloud of suffering feels unsafe for you, it is still effective to use just your thoughts and not your breath to give and receive.

Engaging in giving and receiving will help you shift from fear or resistance to confidence, and to stay present with stability and an open heart. This is significant when there is no other way for you to bring comfort. Using the practice to stay with the suffering you witness is what makes the giving and receiving practice impactful.

Giving and receiving requires trust that you can transform the suffering of another with your attentive, open heart. The practice is not magic. It is based on the essential truth that deep human connection is what brings healing. Giving and receiving practice is not a curative measure, but it does heal by conveying to the one who suffers that they are not alone. Their suffering is held within a greater field of loving presence.

Compassion Is Always Here

In some situations you will choose not to push through the barrier blocking you from extending compassion. This may very likely be the case with resentment/anger but possibly with other barriers as well. Only you can determine the best choice. With certain people or situations, it may take time to come around to extending compassionate action. Just remember that extending compassion is a choice and that offering compassion always feels better than withholding it. I have found it useful to consider how my future self will look back on my decision to either extend or withhold compassion.

As you cultivate your ability to access mindful awareness, it will become easier for you to notice when your compassion is blocked, the first step in moving past compassion barriers. When you notice you are blocked, it becomes easier to come back to your natural compassion. No matter how often your compassion becomes blocked, you can reawaken it again and again.

One of my mother's favorite flowers is the crocus. Where I grew up, they were the first flowers to bloom in the spring. Crocuses, like several other flowers, close at night and reopen with the morning light. Compassion, like the crocus, opens and closes. You can be confident that even when your compassion closes, it won't be long before it opens up again. It may require your time and attention, but the payoff will be worth the effort.

[Practice]

Think about any recent experiences of blocked compassion. Take some time to consider what the barrier was. Ask yourself, "What was the origin of the barrier?" And, "What would it have taken to overcome the barrier?" I encourage you to take the time you need to reflect on these questions and any experiences of blocked compassion, and to write your responses in your journal. Perhaps you can even write a plan for overcoming such barrier(s) in the future. Or write about why you may choose not to work on overcoming the barrier. Stay on the lookout for when your compassion is blocked.

CHAPTER 15

Compassion Is Contagious

This heart of compassion
Radiating with infinite potential
One small act of service
Can change the world

In this chapter you will learn how the benefits of compassion are not limited to the one who extends it and the one who receives it. You will also learn another practice for inspiring compassion.

Ripple Effect

When teaching caregiving courses, I never get tired of sharing with participants one particular aspect of compassion: compassion is contagious. Being aware of this and sharing it with others brings me great joy. The benefits of compassion, including the strengthening of compassionate resolve, are not exclusive to the one who offers and the one who receives. The benefits extend beyond that relationship.

When an act of compassion is witnessed, there are at least three beneficiaries. Certainly, the person who receives the act of compassion benefits. The benefit may include both the decrease in their suffering and the sense of warmth and joy that comes from knowing that someone cared enough to extend compassion.

The person acting with compassion also benefits, because it just feels good to support others. In chapter 9 we talked about the warm glow that follows an act of compassion. This warm glow, processed in the reward or pleasure center of the brain, reinforces our inclination to act compassionately. You could say it strengthens our compassion muscle. Acting compassionately also strengthens one's sense of purpose and meaning. It makes you feel better about yourself.

If a third party observes an act of compassion being extended to someone else, they too will experience a warm glow. In fact, when we witness compassion, the same parts of the brain are activated as when we experience something pleasurable, like a satisfying meal, physical intimacy, or receiving a gift. It is as if the brain thinks we are the direct recipient of compassion when we observe it being received by others.

Moral Elevation

As a caregiver, you can use the compassion contagion to your advantage. That is to say, when you begin to feel like you are tapped out and have no more to give, you can engage in activities that allow you to witness acts of kindness and compassion so as to jumpstart your compassionate resolve. Think of a time when you witnessed firsthand or perhaps through a media source someone doing something nice for someone else. How did observing such an act make you feel? More likely than not, it made you feel pretty good. You probably experienced the warm glow you have been reading about. In 2003 Jonathan Haidt, a social psychologist, coined the term *moral elevation*. He defined it as "a positive emotional state that is described as feeling inspired or moved after witnessing another person perform a remarkable act of virtue."

Experiencing moral elevation is also another way to overcome compassion barriers stemming from negative emotions or mind states such as judgment, anger, fear, anxiety, and disgust. Moral elevation is a positive emotion, and inducing positive emotions helps us overcome the impacts of negative ones. Based on her research looking at the relationship between positive emotions and the duration of negative ones, psychologist Barbara Fredrickson suggests that "positive emotions may loosen the hold that (no longer relevant) negative emotions gain on an individual's mind and body." Researchers are finding that while negative emotions narrow our thinking, positive emotions expand our thinking. Doing something that brings about a positive emotional state helps us to be more creative and more open to taking action.

You can do things to proactively trigger positive emotions. For example, find social media posts depicting people doing kind things for others, take a moment to observe something beautiful in your environment, talk with someone you know who is kind and generous, or think of a time when someone did something kind for you. Doing these sorts of things can evoke moral elevation and help you move beyond negative emotions that may be blocking your compassion or contributing to unhappiness.

It used to be quite common for me to finish a five-hour hospice shift feeling very uplifted and happy. I have come to realize that it was not just because I found deep meaning in the work I was doing or because I experienced the warm glow from offering compassionate action; it was also because I witnessed so much kindness and compassion being expressed by the caregivers around me. After witnessing such admirable behavior, I left each shift with intense and lovely feelings of moral elevation. For me, being in a place where people were in the final days of their lives was anything but depressing; in fact, it was extremely uplifting and healthy. The moral elevation I experienced was simply the byproduct of a hospice culture built around meeting suffering with a clear mind and an open heart.

Whom Do You Elevate?

I invite you to take a moment to consider the people who witness, directly or from afar, your compassionate caregiving. Who are the family members, friends, colleagues, care providers, or strangers who know you are showing up to support someone in need? Now, knowing what it feels like to experience moral elevation from witnessing acts of kindness and compassion, how do you think they are impacted by what they observe in you as a caregiver? Can you allow yourself to acknowledge the benefit these people derive from witnessing you providing care? Let yourself dwell in whatever emotions or thoughts arise for you as you consider the way you impact others in your role. I honestly believe that through your compassion as a caregiver, you are changing the world for the better. The South African theologian Desmond Tutu often shared this encouragement in his speeches and interviews. He is known to have said, "Do your little bit of good where you are; it's those little bits of good put together that overwhelm the world." No matter what form it takes, the way you express your compassion as a caregiver makes a difference. You impact not only the person you are caring for but also the many people around you.

Affirming Your Values

I consider moral elevation to be a form of inspiration. In his beautiful poem "Saint Francis and the Sow," Galway Kinnell reminds us that "sometimes it is necessary to reteach a thing its loveliness." Our loveliness is a reflection of our highest purpose or our most expansive self. It is easy to grow distant from our best self, from our loveliness. Life's difficulties can wear us down, and we can forget that we are capable of acting with virtue for the benefit of others. We can lose contact with how we got here or why we do the things we do. For you, maybe you have lost contact with why you are a caregiver. It may feel like you had no choice, but you always have a choice. You have chosen to stay and not walk away, even when caring for another means sacrificing your freedom and sometimes even your health. When you have lost contact with why you have chosen to be a caregiver, it may be helpful to reteach yourself your loveliness. A beautiful way to do this is through a contemplation known as *values affirmation*, a great way to find inspiration when you most need it.

I would like to share with you the powerful values affirmation inquiry I learned when I was studying to become an instructor of Compassion Cultivation Training. I encourage you to read through the inquiry once and then spend a few moments contemplating the questions below.

- If it is comfortable for you, close your eyes.
- Let your attention find its way to your breath, and rest it there for a few breaths.
- Rest here for however long you need to settle your mind.
- Now imagine yourself resting in a safe place, maybe outdoors looking up at the sky, though someplace comfortable indoors is fine too.
- Without holding back, imagine your highest aspirations, and reflect on the following three questions:
    - If anything were possible, what would I really love to find in my life?
    - If anything were possible, how would I really love to develop as a human being?
    - If anything were possible, what would I really love to offer the world or my community?

How was it for you to consider your responses to these three questions? If you experienced a sense of elevation, notice how that feels in your body. Consider the relationship between your responses to the questions and your role as a caregiver.

A growing body of research shows that reaffirming your core values supports healthy coping with stress, defends against threats to one's self-image, and strengthens a sense of well-being. When you feel good about yourself, you also are more inclined toward behavior that benefits others. So when you notice your compassion decreasing for any reason, it can be helpful to remind yourself of your deepest held values by using the values affirmation inquiry. Do your best to stay in contact with your values. When you lose contact with what is most important to you, remind yourself of your loveliness.

[Practice]

When you notice someone extending compassion, pay attention to how it makes you feel. Note in your body where you feel any emotions arising when you witness compassion being extended to another person. Linger with those feelings for as long as possible.

If you do not have the opportunity to be with people who are extending compassion, seek out such acts through media sources. Notice how watching acts of compassion makes you feel, and dwell in the good feelings that may arise.

If you do not notice anything when watching others express compassion, do not worry. The feelings of moral elevation can be subtle, and if you are not used to tracking such feelings, it may be difficult to notice an impact. Try to let yourself stay curious. The more often you try, the easier it will become to experience the beauty of moral elevation.

LOSS

When you open your heart,
you get life's ten thousand sorrows,
and ten thousand joys.

— Chuang Tzu

Death is a moment-by-moment experience —
we die each moment to the moment.

— Norman Fischer

CHAPTER 16

The Ever-Present Nature of Loss

With each inhale something new arises
With each exhale something falls away
Arising and falling away
This is the nature of things

In this chapter we acknowledge the wide range of losses experienced by both caregiver and care recipient. You will be prompted to consider the types of losses you have experienced and the range of emotions you noticed in response to loss.

Boundless Loss

Outside my window it is early spring, and already the plum tree in the yard is releasing its delicate pink blossoms. The bloom stirs within me a desire to hold onto the beauty of this moment. The joy I feel in the midst of spring is not separate from the sadness I feel for its brevity. And as the plum blossoms thin out, I begin to see beautiful purple leaves emerging in their place.

The plum tree reminds me of the ever-present dance of beginnings and endings, the arising and falling away of all phenomena, which is the nature of our existence. It is simply the way it is. And since loss is an essential part of life, it is an essential part of caregiving. It goes without saying that caring for others entails a wide range of losses. There is the enormous loss that comes with a death, of course, and there are also the smaller, less significant losses that are constant.

It may strike you as counterintuitive, but taking time to consider the impact of loss in your life can have a positive effect on your frame of mind and can enhance your happiness. Although grief may arise, stepping back and contemplating loss and death can also bring feelings of profound gratitude for what is still part of life. Existence and all that animates it becomes more precious, because loss is a reminder of how quickly time passes. In the words of the poet Jeff Foster, "Loss has already transfigured your life into an altar." Loss is a constant reminder that life is worthy of our deepest gratitude.

Caregiving Brings Sacrifice

While you may derive great meaning and satisfaction from caring for someone who needs your support, the role of caregiver, whether or not you chose it, brings with it many changes and sacrifices. Even when embracing the role, there is an opportunity cost to spending time caring for others. There is so much else you could be doing! This kind of loss can bring up a wide range of emotions, each natural and to be expected. For most of the caregivers I have met, it has not been easy to let go of activities, people, objects, identity, or health that they have sacrificed in order to deliver care.

Many family caregivers have shared with me that what they find most difficult is the loss of activities they enjoyed prior to caring for a loved one. Very likely you have put on hold and perhaps lost forever many of the activities that once defined you. Many caregivers simply do not have the time or energy to engage in their favorite activities after spending time caring for a loved one.

For many family caregivers, the responsibility brings with it additional financial burdens that require giving up activities that contribute to relaxation or self-care. One study found that eight out of ten family caregivers report facing regular out-of-pocket costs in the care of their adult loved one. It is reasonable to feel some resentment over spending money that under different circumstances would be spent on your own well-being. And it is natural to feel a sense of loss owing to this type of sacrifice.

It may be that you have stopped reaching out to the people who once brought you joy and a sense of community. Perhaps you don't have time for socializing, or you fear old friends will not be interested in hearing about your responsibilities. Maybe friends stop returning your calls, not knowing what to say or how to show up for you. The more time that passes without contact, the more difficult it can be to pick up the phone and check in. Such isolation and its accompanying sense of loneliness can be a big cause of grief and be extremely detrimental to your well-being.

Shifting Identity

Over time, you may begin to feel like the role of caregiver defines you. For some, this is not a problem. Caregiving is a noble activity and deserving of recognition and admiration. However, some caregivers lament the loss of a lifestyle or an identity that had defined them for much of their lives.

A husband and wife attending one of our Mindful Caregiving Education courses told us about their adult daughter, who was unmarried and had been living on her own before being diagnosed with an advanced debilitating illness. When she became ill, she had no one else to turn to besides her parents, who stepped into the role of caregivers. Though their daughter was not living with them, they spent most of their time caring for her. During the class, the wife tearfully expressed her despair over her daughter's suffering, the unexpected turn of events, and having to give up on the retirement plans she had been looking forward to. "None of my other friends are still taking care of their kids," she shared. It was obvious she loved her daughter and wanted the best for her, but she was finding it difficult to integrate the role of caregiver into her life.

Most of us think of our identity as fixed or unchanging. It is natural to want things to stay the same or to be seen in a particular way. And such desire can be the cause of intense suffering when we cannot let go of our attachment to the way things were or how we want others to view us.

If you have noticed that caregiving has taken a toll on your physical well-being, you are not alone. Twenty-three percent of caregivers in the US report that their caregiving role has had an adverse effect on their health. The responsibilities of caring for a loved one make it difficult to focus on our own well-being. Many caregivers put exercise, diet, sleep, and even maintaining regular visits to the doctor too low on the list of priorities. It can be distressing to step back and think about how much better your health could be if you were not caring for someone. This too is a form of loss.

Emotional Responses to Loss

Of course, not all losses are the same. There are big losses such as the death of a loved one or the end of a primary relationship, and small losses such as losing a favorite article of clothing or having to cancel a date with a friend because you do not feel well. However, many of us recognize default emotional responses or coping patterns, whatever the loss. Grief, a natural response to loss, is multifaceted. Although sadness is the emotion usually associated with grief, it can also stir anger, frustration, confusion, anxiety, and fear. Thinking about your typical emotional response to loss will help you recognize it when you experience it.

Unprocessed grief will leak out sooner or later and is often the root of much of our unskillful behavior, so it helps to be able to identify the underlying emotions triggering any unskillful behavior. I once participated in a communal grief ritual with the wonderful teacher Sobonfu Somé. Sobonfu was an initiated member of the Dagara people in her home country of Burkina Faso. I will never forget the story she told of being confronted at a gas station by a screaming man who accused her of cutting in front of him. She shared with the group her surprise over the accusation and how in the heat of the moment, she asked the man, "Why are you giving me your grief?" Sobonfu understood what was likely going on with the man. It is a shame that he did not. If he had more self-awareness and understanding of his emotions, he likely would have been calmer and more skillful in how he conveyed his anger.

Changing how you respond to the emotions associated with loss requires that you get really curious about what is triggering your emotions. It is much healthier in the long run to stay in contact with the emotions associated with grief rather than denying them or pushing them off for later. This way you can prevent them from controlling your behavior.

Loss is universal, and therefore as a caregiver you will witness the person you are caring for going through loss. This too can potentially activate big emotions. Your emotions can easily get enmeshed in the losses and emotions being experienced by the person you are caring for, especially when they are a family member or a dear friend. If you are caring for a parent, for instance, they may be expressing sadness that there are things they can no longer do. It can be very difficult to separate a parent's sense of loss from your own experience of losing a vibrant, healthy parent. As a caregiver, you are meeting your own loss and showing up as fully as possible for the losses of others. In chapter 19 we will look at how you can prepare yourself emotionally to support someone going through loss and grief. Fully acknowledging the role of loss in your life and tending to your own grief experience is the best preparation for supporting the person you are caring for as they deal with loss. It is never too late to address past loss and grief. Begin right where you are.

[Practice]

Take a few minutes to record in your journal some of the losses you have witnessed recently in the life of the person you are caring for. As you note these losses, consider whether they have had a direct impact on your life. This will of course depend on the nature of your relationship with the person you are caring for. Notice if any strong emotions get activated for you.

- How do you think the person you are caring for is doing with holding their experiences of loss?
- Is there anything more you could do to support them?
- Do you feel any resistance to engaging them in conversation around their loss?

CHAPTER 17

Loss as a Rite of Passage

May I see loss as a teacher
The ordeal of loss
Brings with it wisdom
This wisdom is not mine to keep
It is for those I love

[**This chapter presents a reframing of the loss that is part of caregiving. You will read about the ways the ordeal of loss moves you from one phase of life to the next and how the lessons you acquire in the process can be beneficial to others.**]

I was introduced to the formal practice of contemporary earth-based rites of passage when I was still new to the role of volunteer caregiver. Meeting the hospice physician Scott Eberle changed my life in significant ways. When I first met Scott, he had recently published a book about his own introduction to rites of passage and his experience as the hospice doctor for Steven Foster, who for many years, with his wife Meredith Little, guided rites-of-passage programs for people from all walks of life. While listening to Scott, I had an "aha!" moment. He showed how I could integrate my love for the outdoors with my role of caring for people who were approaching the end of life. It wasn't long before I joined Scott on a rites-of-passage program in Death Valley National Park and began learning this powerful ancient practice. A few years after meeting Scott, and after joining many rites-of-passage programs either as a participant or an assistant, I began guiding others through initiation rites out on the land. (I use the terms rite of passage and initiation interchangeably.)

You may be wondering what rites of passage have to do with your caregiving. Loss and grief are integral parts of being human, and therefore, part of caregiving. And it is impossible to talk about loss and grief without talking about suffering, which plays a central role in any rite-of-passage ceremony. Framing loss and grief as an initiation process helps create meaning and purpose out of the experience. I will explain what traditional rites of passage are and then use them as a framework for discovering how loss and grief can help you grow as a caregiver and enhance the care you provide.

Every culture throughout human history has used initiation rituals to honor and mark the transition from one stage of life to another. The symbolic death/rebirth experience that is part of rites of passage is an essential tool that has supported societies to survive and thrive. Anthropologists have studied rites-of-passage ceremonies in different cultures and find many similarities. Three stages have been identified as part of any initiation: *severance*, *threshold experience*, and *incorporation*.

Severance

Although the person going through the initiation ceremony may be witnessed by guides or community elders, they engage in the process on their own. The individual making their passage must leave their family and community behind to engage in the ceremony. Saying goodbye to who and what you have known up to that point is an essential feature of the symbolic death/rebirth experience. This departure from what is known is the severance phase.

Threshold

The second phase of initiation is the threshold phase, sometimes referred to as the transition phase. This phase is the doorway from one stage of life to another and is marked by suffering. It may entail some great feat of endurance or discomfort. In the rites-of-passage programs I guide, the threshold phase entails being by oneself in a wild place and going without food and comfort for four days and nights. This phase is marked by a threshing or disassembling of who we think we are in the world. It is not easy or comfortable, and that is the point. The more intense or challenging the suffering, the greater the transformation that will be experienced. Different cultures have used different physical challenges as part of their initiation rites.

Incorporation

The third and final phase of initiation is called the incorporation phase. Participants are incorporated back into the body of the community they had said goodbye to. They return as a new person. In some traditional cultures or groups, the person incorporating back into the community would return with a new name. They also return to their community with all the gifts that emerged from the ordeal, which we'll discuss below.

In the context of caregiving, the emotional pain that often characterizes the experience of loss is also an initiation. Profound loss and its accompanying grief can feel very isolating. You may feel like you are completely on your own when you have little time to spend with friends and family. Or friends may abandon you because they cannot relate to what you are going through or they feel uncomfortable in your presence, not knowing what to say or do. Grief differs greatly from person to person. It is easy to feel like no one understands. And it can feel a lot like you have been cut off from your previous life.

As mentioned in chapter 7, the experience of serious illness changes the person who is ill, whether or not they welcome change. Serious illness also changes those who are close to the ailing person. Because illness changes a person and the people around them, there necessarily will be loss. Change and loss go hand in hand. Even though changes may be subtle, the way things were prior to illness is gone. The change you go through when the person you care for is living with a serious illness is a threshold experience.

A caregiver shared in a class that she did not know who she was anymore now that her husband was so weak and confused. She had depended on him for so much before his dementia advanced. She now had to take on more of the household responsibilities as well as care for him. She was figuring out who she was now that things were so different in her life. She was in the process of her identity being dismantled so a new identity could be formed. This is how the threshold phase of initiation works. You are thrust into the ordeal of things falling apart, and you don't really know who will emerge. We sometimes say the threshold phase is the liminal phase during which you are "in between worlds." An old identity is dying, and someone new is being born.

The suffering of the threshold phase can be horrible. I will never forget the night before we took my mother off the machines keeping her alive. Even on life support, my mother was already lost to us. However, the decision to remove her from life support was impossibly difficult. Given the extremely remote chances of a recovery, we decided that letting her die a natural death was the most compassionate action we could take. The decision and the timing of the plan allowed other family members to be at her bedside when she died.

Grief Dismantles the Self

The night before taking my mother off life support was a sleepless night. I cannot remember a more difficult experience. It was impossible to catch up with what was taking place. I had been thrown into the thresher. All night long I cried as I tossed and turned. I could hardly stand to be in my own body or to be with my own mind. I was inconsolable. I had to keep telling myself to surrender to the grief experience. Looking back, I understand what was happening. I was in the death/rebirth phase. I was being reshaped into a person with no mother, and I had no idea how I was supposed to become that person. I was being initiated into the tribe of those who know what it means to lose a parent.

The next day, exhausted, I gathered with my siblings and father at the bedside of my mother to say goodbye. The horrible and beautiful experience of bearing witness as my mother struggled to draw her final breaths didn't last very long. The following days were extremely painful for all of us. I imagine you likely know what this feels like, having had your own experiences of significant loss. Even though I was with my family, I felt very much alone. It helped to have my wife by my side and to be with others in my parents' home, but I experienced how solitary grief can be. Nothing and no one felt familiar during those days.

Whether chronic or acute, resulting from subtle or from significant loss, grief dismantles our sense of self. It challenges our notions of who we are in the world, and it can take a while to reconstruct a new identity. It cannot be rushed. Major grief may be the experience that drives home the reality that identity is at best an illusion. It is not something we can hold onto. It is constantly changing. As we return to routines and relationships, we not only begin to learn who we are now, but we return with gifts born out of the grief experience.

Gifts of the Ordeal

The incorporation phase ideally includes giving away the gifts received from the ordeal of loss and grief. In traditional initiation rites, the one returning to their community shares the realizations or visions they discovered during the threshold phase. They knew their gifts were for the benefit of others and that it would do no good to hold on to them. Giving away the gift might entail taking on a new and important role in the community. Or it might entail sharing an understanding of how some feature of the natural landscape functioned or a different way of approaching a problem. It might simply be to model a new way of behaving that supports the harmony or health of the community.

When caregivers see their ordeal of loss and grief as a rite of passage, the gift they receive from the experience is the wisdom of knowing what it means to be human and to face loss. This is wisdom that others in our society desperately need. Your loved ones and others in your community will face similar loss, and the way you model what you have learned will support them in both subtle and obvious ways.

One thing I try to share with others about what I learned from my mother's death is the benefit of giving yourself over to the grief experience. This entails honest acknowledgment of what emotions are arising and not pushing anything away. I want people to know it is healthiest to let themselves surrender to grief, to grieve fully. There won't be a better time. Give yourself the freedom to feel your grief when it is raw. Even if you must tend to certain responsibilities in the midst of loss, it is vital to find a way to make time for surrendering to grief. I've learned that although grief is powerful and even frightening, it will not destroy you. It will change you from who you knew yourself to be, but you will carry on with life. This is true for all types of loss, not just a major loss like death.

Many of the volunteers who serve with our organization have experienced major loss in their lives. After giving themselves adequate time to fully integrate their loss and process their grief, they show up to support others going through similar experiences. This is one of the ways they give away the gift they have acquired through their grief ordeal.

Zen Caregiving Project occasionally works with a wonderful organization called Imerman Angels. The Imerman model is to recruit people who have come through the experience of living with cancer to be mentors or "angels" to clients who have a new cancer diagnosis. This is a beautiful example of incorporating the initiation experience of battling cancer by supporting others new to the experience.

Ideally, everyone finds a way to give away the gifts they received from struggling through loss. Caregivers are uniquely positioned to do this. By tending to the small losses that are part of caregiving, you become better able to support the person you are caring for with the losses they experience. What have you learned from your experience of losing some of the freedoms you once had? What have you learned from dealing with the loss that comes from witnessing the person you are caring for no longer being able to do the things they once enjoyed?

If you are fortunate enough to live to an old age, you will experience innumerable losses and will at times experience profound grief. Many of the older residents I've met living in hospice have shared that most everyone important to them in life had already died. Most of them had a remarkable quality of ease around their most recent losses. Many of the older men I occasionally meet who lived through the AIDS crisis in San Francisco share that scores of friends and acquaintances died over the course of only a few years. I find that the elders wear their grief like a garment. It becomes part of who they are, always there in subtle ways. The way they carry on with their life despite unimaginable losses is in itself a gift they give to others. When I am in the company of elders, I am reminded that we are defined just as much by our losses as we are by our achievements. And although loss and grief can be extremely painful, it is through these difficult experiences that we acquire crucial insights. We learn to live fully and to help those around us.

[Practice]

Look at the list of losses you recorded in the practice activity in chapter 16. Note three or four of your most significant losses. For each of these, spend some time reflecting on what you have learned from the experiences. Also, consider who might benefit from knowing what you have learned, and think about how you might share what you have learned with those who might benefit.

CHAPTER 18

A Mindfulness-Based Approach to Grief

May I have the courage
To be with what is painful
Moving into each moment
Without knowing what comes next

In this chapter you will learn the usefulness of moving toward your grief and fully acknowledging your authentic experience when grief arises. You will be invited to compose a short intention for how you want to meet the experience of grief.

In the work I do, I often find myself speaking in front of groups of people, sometimes large groups and sometimes small. Like many people, I experience a lot of fear and anxiety when all the focus is on me in a group setting. My body begins to tremble, and I sweat. Sometimes I lose the thread of what I want to say. For much of my life, I thought I could control the fear of being in the spotlight by pushing it aside or pretending that it didn't exist. I hoped no one would notice what I was going through. Looking back, I do not think that approach worked all that well.

Eventually, I learned to befriend fear and to no longer need to push it away. Now I let it be there when it arises. Often I will even name it out loud so others know what I am dealing with; putting it out there feels easier than concealing it. When I welcome the emotion of fear, it no longer gets in my way. I would prefer it didn't arise at all, but it does, so I invite it in like an old familiar friend.

Honest Acknowledgment of Grief

I have found that this mindfulness-based approach also works when it comes to grief. With this approach, you move right up close to the grief. You do not push it away for later or pretend it doesn't exist. As we know by now, mindful awareness is about authenticity and honesty, and it includes everything. So when grief arises, try to acknowledge it fully, and let it be included in your awareness. Even though the experience of grief is unpleasant, you allow it to be there completely because it is what is there for you.

In the previous chapter, I shared the story of my experience the night before my mother was taken off life support. Throughout that long and impossible night, an inner voice kept reminding me to stay with my grief. This voice coached me to get curious and not to turn away. Although it was an awful night, I just kept paying attention to my emotions and did my best to surrender to the experience. Looking back on that night and the days of deep grief that followed, I am grateful I had the wherewithal to coach myself to stay with it. It was extremely painful, yet it was such an essential part of witnessing and honoring my beloved mother in her death. By paying such close attention to each unfolding moment of the experience, I didn't miss a thing. This is just as it should be with such a huge event.

The focus of this chapter is on your grief as a caregiver. What you learn here may be helpful in supporting the person you care for; however, as you read, keep your attention on your own current and past experiences of grief. If you have avoided dealing with grief until now, you might choose to work with the subtle grief that arises from smaller losses. This way, you can gradually build up your capacity to be with profound grief that you may have pushed aside or that you will encounter in the future.

No Rules for Grief

The experience of grief is deeply personal, and it doesn't do much good to compare your grief to anyone else's. While it is supportive to seek companionship when coping with loss, there may be people in your life who will express expectations for how you should deal with your grief. Such expectations, whether conveyed subtly or directly, should be held very loosely. Grief is uncharted territory, and there are no rules or maps for navigating it. So although I am suggesting that you give yourself over to grief, that may not be the right approach for you. Ultimately, you need to decide for yourself what works for you. It is your grief experience.

Turning toward grief requires trust — trust that eventually you will emerge on the other side where life after loss will become the new normal and the emotions of grief will settle down. Just as there is no road map for grief, there is no timeline. For you, it will take as long as it takes to reach the place where you are not overwhelmed by grief. Giving yourself the time you need to let grief run its course is not always easy. We live in a fast-paced culture that really does not support taking adequate time for grieving. You may perceive pressure from work, friends, even family to "get on with it." Nonetheless, I hope you can give yourself permission to resist this kind of pressure and let your grief take as long as it takes. Grief is deeply personal, and it is for you to decide how long is too long. While grieving may take a long time, if it interferes with essential activities in your life or if feelings of overwhelm persist, it may be necessary to seek the support of a therapist. In chapter 23, I offer some ways to overcome the typical time constraints of daily life that may limit your ability to attend to your grief.

The Many Faces of Grief

Grief manifests in a variety of ways. While sadness is the emotion most often associated with grief, it is not the only one. You may shut down emotionally, or you may have outbursts. Whatever form it takes, you may find yourself in the midst of grief when you least expect it. Grief can take more energy than you will be ready to give it. Yet even so, pushing grief away only works for so long before it catches up with you.

Despite the difficulty of grief, like all struggles, it brings gifts. Recently, a friend who has been in a long-term relationship that ended described his time of grief as a time of awakening, a chance to reacquaint himself with what matters to him most. Grief is an opportunity to come back to one's true self. Francis Weller writes beautifully about this in his book *The Wild Edge of Sorrow*: "To honor our grief, to grant it space and time in our frantic world, is to fulfill a covenant with soul — to welcome all that is, thereby granting room for our most authentic life." Grief will return you to your most authentic life if you let it, if you give it your full attention.

Building Capacity to Be with Loss

Turning away from loss and grief for whatever reason puts off the inevitable. Grief will show up one way or another. If you give it your attention and let it be just as it is, you will build your capacity to be with loss. The lessons you learn from your grief, whether it is born out of small or profound losses, prepares you for future loss. Building your capacity to be with the loss experience does not mean you will not feel the pain of grief in the future. It only means you will have a frame of reference. You will know that you can give yourself over to grief without it destroying you. You will know that there is an alternative to pushing grief away.

Self-compassion plays an important role in the experience of grief. You will recall that the first of the three components of self-compassion is recognizing that you are suffering. Giving your full attention to grief means you are honest with yourself about your struggle and discomfort. This recognition is an admission of your vulnerability.

The vulnerability of grief is universal. When we are in the depths of our grief, knowing that others also experience it may bring little solace in the short term. However, as time passes, we may find comfort from remembering that we are not alone in our pain. Loss and grief are part of our shared humanity.

After my mother died and I emerged from the period of overwhelming grief that disrupted all aspects of my life, I felt I had joined the vast community of people who knew what it meant to no longer have a mother. This was both saddening and reassuring. It brought comfort by reminding me that I would be okay. The universe has held those of us who have lost mothers for as long as there have been mothers.

There is a deeply moving story about grief that has been told since the time of the historical Buddha. To me, it speaks to the essential role of acknowledging shared humanity in the experience of loss and self-compassion. In the story, a young woman named Kisa Gotami seeks the Buddha after the death of her newborn child. She is overcome with grief and begs this powerful teacher to bring her only child back to life. The wise one tells her that if she can bring him a single mustard seed from a household that has not known the pain of loss, he would restore the infant to life.

Kisa Gotami searched her village and beyond for a family that had not known loss. Each person she spoke to offered her comforting words to ease her broken heart, but none gave her the mustard seed she was seeking. On her search, Kisa Gotami found communion in her loss with others who knew the kind of grief she was holding. She returned to the Buddha empty-handed and still full of grief but knowing she was not alone.

The Buddha's assignment offered Kisa Gotami the compassion she had to learn for herself. When grief leaves us crazy and inconsolable, sooner or later we must find our way to self-compassion. If we are going to surrender to the grief experience, we must be able to fully acknowledge our suffering, we must remember we are not alone, and we must hold our experience with kindness. This is how we endure without denying our authentic experience.

Identifying Default Approaches to Grief

As you have been reading along, have you thought about how you have dealt with your own grief? In the many years of working in the end-of-life and caregiving arena, I have come to observe that people have particular default attitudes and behaviors when it comes to experiencing grief. In a caregiver training my wife participated in, she shared that when grief begins to arise, she makes herself busy with house cleaning, a coping mechanism. Another caregiver shared that he loses himself in a work project. Others look for things to make them happy. Others still will find a creative outlet to channel the emotional experience. The style of grieving that includes getting busy with a task requiring thought rather than emotional processing is normal and in psychology literature is known as "instrumental grieving."

Once you have identified your default approach to grief, check in with yourself and ask if it is the healthiest way to integrate grief into your life. You may decide you want to try a new approach. Setting an intention for how you want to show up for grief is a great place to begin. In the practice activity below, take some time to think about how you want to show up for your grief. Who do you want to be in the experience of grief? You will be guided to compose a short statement that can be kept nearby to inspire you in the face of grief.

Like Kisa Gotami, who desperately tried to find a household untouched by loss, you have likely learned that loss and grief are an inevitable part of being human. No one is untouched by the emotional pain that accompanies loss. It is never too late to change how you show up for the experience of grief. It begins with the desire to cultivate self-awareness and a willingness to change. Then you might try a new approach. Take your time, be gentle with yourself, and remember that only you know what is best for you.

[Practice]

You will know grief again and again. What is your intention for the next time grief arises? Write down a short intention for how you will meet the experience. You might form your intention as a "May I…" statement or a "Let me…" statement.

Once you have written down your grief intention, keep it in a place where you will see it when you need it. Take a photo with your phone, and save it to its own album so it is easy to locate. If helpful, you might send it to a trusted friend or family member so you have a kind witness to remind you.

Remember, intentions are not rules you must follow. They are reminders of what you are capable of doing. They are sources of inspiration. They support you to be your biggest, most courageous self.

CHAPTER 19

Supporting Others with Their Loss

With a compassionate heart as my guide
I invite you to take my hand
I will accompany you through loss

As a caregiver you are uniquely positioned to support the person you are caring for as they experience loss in all its forms. In this chapter, you will learn ways to help ease the natural process of loss experienced by anyone living with illness.

I think it is fair to say that we live in a society that does not support a healthy relationship to impermanence. Most of us do not want to think about our own mortality or how we relate to the experience of loss. We might even describe mainstream culture as being death-phobic. The influence of mainstream media and mass marketing has contributed to an obsession with youth and a negative view of the normal aging process, which can make us think that loss and death are unnatural. And this resistance to accepting impermanence and change causes unnecessary suffering for those living with illness.

Addressing Spiritual Needs

If you are a caregiver courageous enough to see that the person you are caring for is more than their illness, you are well suited to offer support that extends beyond their medical or physical needs. Acknowledging the losses that come with the illness places the person you are caring for directly within the realm of spirit. Turning toward loss provides an opening for considering the larger spiritual context of their experience. As a caregiver, you can play an important role in addressing the spiritual needs of the one(s) you care for.

I view the realm of spirit as a place of mystery that unfolds moment to moment, a place where there are no clear answers. However, for some, spiritual or religious beliefs offer clarity regarding life's biggest questions, such as why we suffer and how we find meaning when living with illness. What you believe to be true may not be useful for the person you are caring for, and it may be most supportive to offer questions that allow them to find their own answers. Finding answers that address life's biggest challenges is most productive when there is a witness or someone to talk with. You can be that witness. You can be that conversation partner.

Always Dying to Things

As you deepen your practice of cultivating present-moment awareness and attuning to loss, you will begin to notice that nothing stays the same for long. Every aspect of our lives is touched by change and impermanence. This truth may cause some uneasiness, but only if you lose sight of how tightly intertwined loss is with new beginnings. It is impossible to imagine a world without loss.

The familiar phrase "this too shall pass" includes both the good and the bad, and I find this reassuring. While it may be painful to say goodbye to certain parts of life, perhaps we can acknowledge the upside of impermanence. I am sure you have experienced great relief when an uncomfortable situation ends. Think of sitting in a dentist's chair. How wonderful it is when the dental work ends and you can walk out of the office. When I was very ill a few years ago and in constant pain, reminding myself that one way or another the pain would eventually subside was one of the few things that brought me solace. Nothing seemed to help me but the acknowledgment of impermanence. Even some deaths bring with them a profound sense of relief. The intense suffering we may witness as someone is dying can be alleviated only with the drawing of the final breath.

So much of what is dear to you and part of your life exists because something was given up to make space for it. If we did not experience loss, nothing new would ever happen. No new discoveries, accomplishments, or adventures. No births. I am sure you get the point. Acknowledging the necessity of impermanence does not mean there is anything wrong with feeling the grief that accompanies loss. We can recognize that loss is simply part of life and still grieve our losses. In his book *Awareness*, the Jesuit spiritual teacher Anthony De Mello writes, "We're always dying to things. We're always shedding everything in order to be fully alive and to be resurrected at every moment." "Always dying to things" is another way of saying that we are constantly changing. Embracing this constant change is how we can live fully, including acknowledging the truth of grief when it arises.

When talking about how to best support the person you are caring for with their loss and grief, it is useful to acknowledge that there are different kinds of losses and degrees of intensity. Losses subtle and profound have transformative effects. Obviously, losing one's freedom to spend time socializing with friends will impact you differently than the death of your loved one. A woman who was a caregiver to her husband attended a grief support session and explained that she no longer knew who she was since her husband's death. This is a common feeling for those who have experienced profound loss, like the death of a life partner. She was in the early stages of figuring out who she was now as she formed new relationships. The smaller chronic losses you and the person you are caring for experience throughout the illness journey cannot be compared to the major loss that a death represents. However, small losses, if not acknowledged and given their due, will over time accumulate and can build into intense grief.

As a caregiver you will observe the wide range of loss and grief in the person you are caring for. The way you offer emotional support will of course depend on the severity of the grief you witness. Whether the person you are caring for is experiencing mild or intense grief, you will be most supportive if you have taken some time to examine your own relationship to loss and grief.

Knowing Your Own Story of Loss

Our hospice volunteer training at Zen Caregiving Project emphasizes the importance of deeply exploring one's own relationship to impermanence, loss, and death. We have found that this exploration is necessary for caregivers before showing up to support people living with chronic or terminal illness who are experiencing intense constant loss and grief. If a volunteer is going to sit at the bedside of someone experiencing profound loss, we want to know that they have looked at their own relationship to grief and considered the reality of their own eventual death. We want the volunteer caregivers to become intimate with the thoughts and emotions that arise when thinking about past, current, and future losses. Otherwise, we cannot be sure that witnessing a grieving patient won't trigger destabilizing emotions that can interfere with the support they provide or their general sense of well-being. We want to know that the volunteer will be available to tend to the person they are serving rather than having to tend to their own emotional needs. We want to know that they have the capacity to grieve deeply and have become familiar with their own emotional processing in the face of loss.

When teaching our courses to paid and family caregivers, our instructors encourage the same personal exploration of emotions and attitudes toward loss and impermanence. Thinking about past and future losses can be uncomfortable. However, spending time in this territory is essential to providing steady emotional and spiritual support to a loved one, patient, or client living with chronic or serious illness. I invite you to take a moment or two to step back and consider whether you have spent adequate time truly thinking about how you relate to the losses you have experienced and your own mortality.

You might consider these questions:

- Do I avoid thinking about loss?
- Do I think I have adequately grieved the losses I have experienced?
- Am I comfortable thinking or talking about my own aging, sickness, and death?
- What is my story of loss?

If you conclude that you have not given enough attention to the presence of loss in your life, you are not alone. I would venture that most people have not spent adequate time thinking about these things. You may be asking what the relationship is between cultivating intimacy with your emotions and attitudes toward loss and the care you provide to others. The emotional support you provide to someone when they are grieving improves as you become more comfortable thinking and talking about loss and grief. If you don't give yourself the opportunity to think about your story of loss, and to experience the accompanying emotions, it is very likely that you will find it difficult to show up for the big emotions that may arise as the person you care for shares their grief.

When encountering grief, you may find your emotions become enmeshed with the emotional experience of the person you are caring for, especially when that person is a family member. What you see or hear may remind you of your own losses. The loss you witness may have a direct impact on your own life, or you may simply be deeply moved by the poignancy of the loss you witness. Being familiar with your own grief emotions and your own story around loss can help you maintain emotional stability so you can be fully present for the one you are caring for.

When you intimately know your own story of loss and grief, your openhearted presence will be unobscured by unstable emotions. As you get to know your loss story deeply, you learn to recognize when strong emotions or thoughts begin to arise. Emotions may arise, but they are familiar and no longer debilitating or even distracting. Awareness of your emotional patterns allows you to be more available for inviting the person you support to go wherever they need to go to truly honor their grief experience. If you are unfamiliar or afraid of your emotions, you won't invite others to fully express theirs. This avoidance, whether subtle or obvious, will be very limiting for the person you are caring for.

Sadly, it is common for people living with chronic or serious illness to have to shift from receiving emotional support to providing support for family members or others who are overwhelmed by emotions. When a person receiving care pivots to offer emotional support to others, it denies them the opportunity to process their own grief and arrive at a place of peace with their circumstances. Ideally, the person you are caring for is able to process their grief with the support of others around them — and this is not possible when those around them are overwhelmed by their own emotions.

Emotional Resonance

I am not suggesting that you as a caregiver should not experience or express your emotions. Often, I experience emotional resonance with someone who is feeling profound grief, and sometimes this resonance includes tears. Such emotional expression is the experience of empathy we considered in earlier chapters. However, I have worked with my own grief territory enough to recognize, with or without tears, if I am getting too close to emotional collapse or becoming thoroughly overwhelmed by emotions.

I used to point out to our volunteers and nurses that it was okay to cry with a dying resident, just not to cry louder than them or their family members. This was my way of saying that emotional expression is okay, even welcomed, but emotional collapse is not useful. Although it may be very challenging for family caregivers, I recommend not depending on the person you are caring for to support you with big emotions. If you are prone to emotional collapse when witnessing another's grief, very likely you have experienced a loss that you have not explored deeply enough.

You are likely familiar with stories of people who die once the family members have left the room. I have observed this happening fairly often. I believe that part of the reason this happens is that the person who is dying does not want to be the cause of sadness for their loved ones. For people living with an illness, whether it is terminal or chronic, witnessing and holding the emotional experience of those around them is burdensome. It is a blessing for someone receiving your care to know that you have developed the skills to maintain emotional stability. Such stability conveys your support, something that cannot be faked. You can express your love and your grief without it becoming a distraction when the focus should be on the person experiencing the grief that illness or even death brings.

People dealing with long-term chronic or serious illness are extremely sensitive to the energy of others. This is especially true when a person receiving care is confined to their bed. Their world gets very small, and they are finely attuned to what is going on around them. With this kind of sensitivity, it is not possible to fake how you are feeling emotionally. To avoid the need to fake it, you can cultivate your mindful awareness and use the skills you have learned to become deeply familiar with strong emotions and the thoughts that trigger them. Spending time getting intimate with your grief story will mean you will never have to avoid or fake how you are truly feeling. You will be able to fully experience your grief and provide a steady presence for the one you are caring for.

While it may not be possible for you to do anything to cure the illness of the person you are caring for, you can do a great deal to make it safe for them to meet and process their grief. Supporting another through their experience of loss may not be easy, but it can be one of the most important parts of the caregiver role. Facing loss directly takes courage. Turning toward loss and grief with the person you are caring for is deep soul work and can clarify what is most important in life. The spiritual teacher Ram Dass had a phrase that beautifully characterizes this type of emotional and spiritual support. He said that in this journey through life, "we're all just walking each other home." Whatever home means to the person you are caring for, I hope your walk with them includes a willingness to turn toward loss and grief.

[Practice]

Spend ten to fifteen minutes writing down the various losses you have experienced throughout your life. You might organize them into the following categories:

- **People who once were in your life**. These can include both those close to you, such as a spouse/partner, child, or close friend as well as the people you encounter as part of your daily routine, such as the postal carrier, the grocery store clerk, a neighbor. (Don't forget to include animal companions.)
- **Activities you once engaged in regularly**. This could be anything, like walking the dog, playing tennis, knitting, or reading a book.
- **Roles you played.** These roles could include being a daughter or son, a sibling, a teacher, a friend, or a runner.
- **Objects that once were important to you**. Maybe this is a home, your eyeglasses, a favorite piece of jewelry or clothing, or a car.
- **Physical features or abilities.** You could include hearing, vision, running, your hair, your legs.

As you record your losses, be sure to check in with yourself and notice any changes in physical sensations, emotions, and thoughts. If strong emotions arise during this practice, take a moment to rest attention on physical sensations, identifying where the emotions are showing up in your body.

CHAPTER 20

Inviting Conversations About Loss

When ready, bring whatever you need to say
Trust my attentive ear and my open heart
I will hold your story

[**Inviting conversations about loss is an essential part of caregiving. This chapter will help prepare you for discussing loss, an inevitable part of living with illness, with the person you are caring for.**]

The last time I visited with my maternal grandmother before she died, one thing was very clear: "Bubbe Sylvia" wanted to talk about her approaching death. She had experienced a lot of difficulty in her life, and it was impossible for her to discuss what it meant to die without talking about her other losses. My grandfather, Roy, died at a young age, and Sylvia raised her two daughters on her own. She lived with a chronic autoimmune disorder, myasthenia gravis, for about twenty years, preventing her from doing many of the things she once enjoyed. Her speech was impacted, and she tired easily. The illness also altered her appearance by causing her right eyelid and part of her mouth to droop. Sylvia had a very difficult relationship with her two adult daughters. And in her early eighties, Sylvia moved from the Detroit area, where she had lived her entire life, to Portland, Oregon, to be near my aunt and her family, and she deeply missed the place she had grown up in. While the details may differ, my grandmother's losses are not unlike those faced by many people who reach their eighties. And, like others living with long-term chronic illness, she wanted her story of loss witnessed by someone she trusted. I will always cherish the time I spent listening to whatever stories she wanted to share. I trust that it brought Bubbe Sylvia solace knowing that I had a sense of her suffering and that her stories would live on in me.

Discussing Losses Big and Small

Getting comfortable with conversations about loss is relevant in the context of both long-term illness, when death may be many years in the future, and serious illness that may result in death relatively soon. Even if the person you are caring for has many years of life remaining, including end-of-life priorities in conversations about loss will better prepare them and others around them for when that time comes. May the death of the person you are caring for be in the distant future; however, it is never too early to begin thinking about how to prepare for death.

Ideally, you will have spent adequate time with your own story of loss and grief, as discussed in the last chapter. Knowing your own story intimately will make it easier for you to set it aside and be fully attentive to the story of the person you are caring for. Conversations about loss with someone who is living with illness often entail a lot of listening. This does not mean there will never be an opportunity for you to share your thoughts on what it means to experience loss; however, you will be most supportive if you do not urgently need to have your own story heard when the topic of loss comes up in conversation.

I am extremely fond of the metaphor used by hospice physician Scott Eberle when talking about supporting people who are at the end of their life or experiencing profound loss. Scott views the activity of holding space for story as presenting a vessel or bowl to the person sharing their story. He suggests that knowing your own story of loss and grief intimately allows you to be at ease with emptying your bowl so you can fill it with another's story. Having spent numerous hours with Scott as he listens to others' stories, I see that the vessel he offers has limitless capacity to hold a story. It is truly an act of generosity that helps deepen the storyteller's understanding of their experience. Scott's way of listening is good medicine; it both lightens the burden of the storyteller and helps them see their life in a new way.

Getting to know your own story of loss and grief will allow you to develop ease with discussing the topic. Your willingness to talk about your own losses will offer an invitation to others to talk about their losses and their eventual death. I have come to believe that most people are very open to discussing loss when they feel safe with someone who can meet them in the conversation. Recently, I met with a group of grief counselors for a large hospice, and one counselor shared something that I have also found to be true. As soon as an acquaintance learns that you work in the field of loss and grief or are at ease with the topic, they bring their stories. Your willingness to share from a place of authenticity and vulnerability invites others to discuss loss, often a hard topic to discuss.

In a conversation with the grief counselors, a social worker shared a moving story about meeting with a client who had recently experienced the death of a sibling. Despite the social worker's attempts to engage her, the woman was very reluctant to open up about her grief. The social worker decided to share with her client that she too had experienced the death of a sibling not so long ago and what it was like for her to be in profound grief. Once the client heard that the social worker had a loss story similar to hers, she opened up about how she was coping. The two were able to connect deeply around their shared vulnerability of being human beings experiencing grief.

There is growing recognition that loss, an unavoidable part of life, must be talked about more often. It has been satisfying to see the emergence of a wider public conversation about loss, death, and grief. There are a number of organizations like ours that are doing great work changing attitudes about these essential topics and providing a space to discuss them. End Well hosts an annual symposium in which thought leaders and cultural influencers share their experiences of profound loss. Zen Caregiving Project regularly hosts a forum to discuss perspectives on loss and death, which we call Open Death Conversations. Death Over Dinner, Death Cafe, and the Dinner Party each offer resources to anyone interested in hosting a conversation about loss and death. Reimagine sponsors a variety of events in person and online that encourage us all to reimagine our individual and collective relationship to death and dying. The Conversation Project provides resources for discussing with friends and loved ones your wishes for care through the end of life. These are just a few examples of what is available to support you in getting comfortable discussing loss, death, and grief. Please see the resources section at the back of the book for more information about these organizations.

Meeting Others Where They Are

Even if you are comfortable talking about loss, it does not mean the person you are caring for will be. You may be open to hearing their burdensome thoughts and feelings about grief, and yet they refuse to go there. You cannot force someone to talk about something they do not want to talk about. If you find yourself in this situation, there are things you can say and do to help the person you are caring for feel safer sharing.

I tried for almost twenty years to draw my mother into a meaningful conversation about end-of-life issues. Each time I tried to bring up the topic, she would get upset and tell me she just couldn't discuss such things. I started to feel as if I was inflicting pain on her, definitely not something I wanted to do. In some of those attempts at conversation, my father, who seemed more willing to discuss the topic, would try to put it off as a way to protect my mother from experiencing any emotional pain. My mother held profound grief from the death of her father at a young age and the neonatal death of her fourth child, my newborn sister. Her deep grief would show up in a variety of unexpected ways, but she did her best to avoid addressing it directly.

Ultimately, I had to accept my mother's resistance to talking about her losses or her wishes for end-of-life care. I continued to try different approaches, all to no avail. In the end, when she was suddenly dying, we did not know what her end-of-life wishes were. We made some assumptions based on her attitudes toward the topic, but it would have been easier for our family had she been able to find her way to discussing the topic before her death. In the next chapter we will look more closely at end-of-life wishes and advanced medical directives.

When you detect resistance, rather than going straight to the topics of loss, death, and grief, you might begin by engaging the person you are caring for with questions about change. This allows you to test the waters to see how open they are to this kind of conversation. For instance, someone who has been living with chronic illness may be willing to talk about what has changed for them since becoming ill, even though they do not want to talk about their grief or what may happen if they do not get better. Or they may be willing to talk about how they felt during times of meaningful transition in their life like a birth, a graduation, a wedding, retirement, or the end of a friendship. Talking about changes can be a gateway to deeper conversations that directly address losses, grief, and even end-of-life wishes. The key is meeting people where they are and not rushing them to open up. I also encourage you to let go of any attachment to particular outcomes for the conversations.

Availability Is a Form of Service

With some people, the most you will be able to do is let them know that you are available to talk when they are ready. While you can verbalize this, the person you are caring for may be able to pick up on your receptivity without your even saying a word. The more you strengthen your mindfulness and compassion, the more you will be seen as receptive to difficult conversations. Others will notice your calm, your open heart, and your attention. They will recognize your emotional stability as your willingness to meet whatever comes your way. Your availability for difficult conversations is a profound form of care. Do not underestimate the benefit of others knowing that you are receptive to conversations about loss and grief, even if they do not engage you in such conversations.

Just because the person you are caring for does not want to talk about difficult subjects now does not mean they won't feel different later — even later on the same day. One caregiver who attended a support group session recently explained that her father was open to talking about his losses in the morning, but later in the day, he would not go there. She did not know how to make sense of this; however, she learned to invite him to talk about loss only in the mornings. You may need to be patient and wait for the right moment.

The Right Person at the Right Time

If you are a family caregiver, it could be that the person you are caring for would like to talk about their loss and grief — just not with you. Although this may be painful to accept, it should be respected. This is often true for people caring for a parent. In families, roles and patterns of communication are often firmly established. Some family members may find expressing the kind of vulnerability that is often part of a deep conversation about loss unacceptable. Some parents, when experiencing moments of heightened emotions or what they perceive as weakness, do not want this to be seen by their kids. On the other hand, I have heard from people living with serious illnesses that their adult kids do not want to hear any talk of end-of-life wishes or how they are feeling about the losses they are experiencing. When it comes to communication, family dynamics are often complicated. If it is too uncomfortable to raise the topic, I hope there is someone you can reach out to who can have such a conversation with the person you are caring for.

Maria attended one of our family caregiver courses just as we began offering them several years ago. After completing the course,

Maria reached out to me to share a story about her father, whom she was caring for. During a drive to a medical appointment, her father expressed that he was feeling depressed because there was so much he could no longer do. Her father's sadness made Maria feel uncomfortable, and she began trying to cheer him up by redirecting him to a different, more uplifting topic. Later, on reflection, she realized that she had denied her father the opportunity to talk about his sadness and the changes in his life. He really did not have anyone else he could talk to. At her next opportunity, she apologized and invited her father into a conversation about how he was feeling. Maria shared that it ended up being a very rich conversation and brought her and her father closer. Maria was grateful that even if it was after the fact, she realized what she had done and was able to correct it.

The Invitation

Mindful awareness helps you to notice when the person you are caring for is having a big emotional experience. When you notice this, you might try saying, "You seem to be going through something. Can you describe how you are feeling?" It may be difficult for the person you are caring for to describe their emotions, but this can be a very good place to start. If they have difficulty describing their emotions, you could ask where in their body they experience them. If you are perceived as calm and attentive, it is more likely that the other person will share more about what is true for them, even if it takes time. Even if it is difficult to describe exactly what they are feeling, they may begin to reveal the thoughts triggering their emotions.

A great way to enter into a conversation about loss is to pull out photo albums. Having a photo to talk about helps both parties get beyond the initial barrier of not knowing where to begin. Looking at old photos with the person you are caring for is an important conversation starter at every stage of illness. It is especially helpful if the person you are caring for is approaching the end of their life.

Life Review

An essential feature of the end-of-life experience or major life transitions is the life review activity. Life review is the process of looking back over one's life and telling stories of important events, activities, and relationships. It is often the last opportunity for a person to reflect on their life before saying goodbye to it. As a caregiver, you can play an important role in facilitating this process. Doing a life review is how we humans make peace with how we have lived. Telling life review stories allows the reviewer to celebrate the joys and successes of life and to feel gratitude for what they have experienced. And it offers an opportunity to reflect on how they have dealt with failures and disappointments or perhaps on how they are still holding these experiences. It is a time to think about the relationships that have filled one's lifetime. Sharing life review stories can loosen the attachment to all that is being lost.

The life review process can, for some, be filled with big emotions. Thinking about the good stuff can be pleasant. However, thinking about the difficult and messy stuff can be painful. As a caregiver you are in a position to encourage self-forgiveness when the person you are caring for expresses regret for some mistake or transgression. It is possible you may be the person who has been wronged. If so, you may see an opportunity to offer forgiveness. Forgiveness is not always an easy thing to grant; however, this is another case where it may be helpful to think of your future self. Long after the person you are caring for has died, will you regret not expressing forgiveness when you had the chance?

In the life review process, most people identify relationships that did not end well. Unresolved issues in a relationship can weigh heavily on someone approaching death. As a caregiver, you may be able to facilitate communication between the person you are caring for and the person with whom they have unfinished business. This could be in the form of a letter that you help write, which may or may not be sent. Or perhaps you assist them with a phone call. If direct contact is not possible or desired, you may be able to stand in as a surrogate. Perhaps you can ask, "If that person were here with you now, what would you say to them? Let me be that person." In the role of surrogate, you might even offer resolution with, "Please forgive me." Or, "I forgive you." This can bring solace to someone who regrets not saying what needed to be said when they had the opportunity.

You will likely notice that the person you are caring for reaches a point when they are feeling complete with the life review process, no longer needing to look back. I remember spending time with Benny, a man in his late eighties who was living at our guest house. His wife Benita was outgoing and extremely clever. She was very attentive to Benny and his needs. Benny was a quiet man, and Benita noticed that he did not have much to say to staff or volunteers. She brought some photo albums to leave in Benny's room so he would have something to talk about. Benny was very comfortable answering questions about the photos that went way back and began telling his life review stories. Then one day when I was spending time with Benny I pulled out one of the photo albums to energize our lagging conversation. He waved away the album and shared that he no longer wanted to talk about the photos. It became obvious to me and to others that Benny was done with that activity. He lived another couple of weeks. During that time he seemed at ease just sitting quietly with others. Benny struck me as a man who was ready for whatever came next.

Hope

When you invite conversations about loss, the person you are caring for may express hope for a cure of their condition. Hope is an essential feature of living with an illness. It helps keep people engaged with life even when it becomes difficult due to illness. Hope can become a way of coping with overwhelming difficulty. While you may want to avoid crushing hope, I encourage you to also avoid perpetuating false or unrealistic hope. Hope is always focused on the future and may prevent the person you are caring for from reaching a place of acceptance for what is here and now. As a caregiver, it is a fine line to walk.

For people living with a terminal illness, false hope can cause them to be surprised by their own death and deny them and those around them the opportunity to prepare. When we are not comfortable talking about loss and death, hope can be a convenient escape from the reality of what is truly happening. Stephen Jenkinson, a writer and teacher who has spent many years working with people who are dying, wrote in his book *Die Wise*, "Hope almost always makes sure that it is too late to learn how to die for dying people in a death-phobic culture." I once heard him say, "Hope is the enemy of a good death." This is a controversial statement but worth considering. What you consider a good death may not be a good death for the person you care for. Nonetheless, determining what the person you are caring for considers a good death will only emerge through conversation, and hope may interfere with having this conversation.

I have witnessed families in hospice keenly focused on the possibility of a miracle. No one wants to give up on their loved one, so this is understandable. Yet these families often miss the opportunity for closure, to say the things they often later wish they had said. I believe that hope for a miracle must be balanced with conversations that support a dying person to share what they need to say before it is too late. In some religions and cultures, the idea of miracles holds an important place, and I mean no disrespect to these belief systems. I think there can be both a wish for a miracle and an acknowledgment of what is really happening. I find no harm in engaging a dying person in honest conversations about loss and their end-of-life wishes while also praying together for a miracle.

Understanding Is Overvalued

Conversations about loss are more than just the words shared. Many of us are attached to understanding the meaning of what others have to say. I have noticed that when people are nearing the end of their lives, they often speak in metaphors, a type of code they use to convey their fears, curiosity, or assumptions about what is about to happen. I believe finding clarity when we do not fully understand what is being shared is less important than simply listening and paying attention. I once sat with a man who was approaching his death when he asked which way he should go when he reached the top of the stairs. I told him I thought he would be safe going either left or right, and he seemed reassured by my response. I have sat with many people at the end of their life who expressed a desire to go home. I think this is about returning to a sense of comfort or belonging and less about a particular place. When you hear something surprising, do not be too quick to take what is shared literally.

Some people experiencing serious illness or dementia express themselves in ways that do not make logical sense. Although someone may have lost their ability to communicate clearly, it is likely they can still process emotions. If you are caring for someone who expresses themselves unclearly, you can listen for the energy or emotion behind the words rather than trying to make sense of what they are saying. In this type of situation, openhearted presence is most important. Sharing that you do not understand what they are trying to say may be distressing to them and most likely will not lead to greater clarity. Interpreting what is being said is less supportive than listening attentively or conveying that you are there for them. You might respond by addressing the emotion you detect behind the words with gentle reassurance.

I have very fond memories of Charles, whom I met while volunteering. Each week I looked forward to visiting this man who radiated a kind of brightness. A tall man with a head of thick white hair and a big smile, he never appeared distressed by his dementia. I recall sitting with him in the great room on the palliative care floor of the San Francisco County long-term-care hospital, Laguna Honda Hospital. Charles shared lengthy stories with me. Though I could understand the individual words he spoke, when those words were strung together, I could make no meaning out of them. However, what was really wonderful was the way his facial expressions and hand gestures revealed clues about his story and his personality. His nonverbal messages told me he was a playful, even mischievous raconteur. They helped me know when to laugh and when to tune in carefully. When I needed to move on, I would excuse myself by thanking him for his story. He always seemed happy to have shared it with me. Maybe I was deceiving him by letting him believe I understood his stories, but I trust he felt seen and sensed a connection. Ultimately, that seemed most important.

Death Lodge

Years ago I was fortunate to be introduced to an ancient practice that has supported me greatly ever since. This is the practice of the "death lodge." The death lodge is a stage in preparing for death and can be found historically, in some form, in cultures around the world. In many tribal communities, when someone knew they were dying, they would place themselves on the edges of the community or village and begin to retreat. Moving into the death lodge phase sent a message that the community member was preparing for the end, and friends and family were invited to say goodbye. Once saying goodbye to relations, the dying person moved on to a conversation with themselves about their life, continuing the life review process on their own.

I would like to share a story of a crucial experience in my life to explain the five essential statements that guide the death lodge conversation. Several years ago, one of my closest friends, David, decided to move his family to Europe so he and his wife could pursue new work. I met David during my first year of college, and over the years he has become like a brother to me. As his departure date approached, I knew I had to mark this big change in my life. We planned an overnight backpacking trip to circumambulate our beloved Mt. Tamalpais. I told him I had a ritual planned for us that I would share with him at some point during the hike.

On the second day of hiking we paused on a wooded knoll overlooking a beautiful valley. I opened by telling David I had things to say. I reminded him of the death lodge conversation I had once told him about and explained that I needed to have such a conversation with him, even though it was likely that neither of us was dying any time soon and that we would see each other again. He agreed, and after joking around a bit to make light of the sadness we were both feeling, we began.

First I said to him, *I forgive you*, and I elaborated on a few things he had done over the years that I found hurtful. Then I asked him to *please forgive me* for anything I had done that may have caused him hurt or anger. Then I told him that I *love* him and how important our friendship is to me. This led me to an expression of *gratitude*, thanking him for his friendship and his role in my life. I ended with saying *goodbye*. Rather than elaborate on the details of the conversation, I will share the essence of the death lodge conversation: *Please forgive me. I forgive you. I love you. Thank you. Goodbye.* If these statements can be shared authentically, the relationship is made whole and there is closure. Each person knows how the other feels, and nothing more needs to be said. I knew that if I never saw David again, there would be no unfinished business.

Though neither of us was actually dying, we were honoring the symbolic death that his move represented. We were saying goodbye to one phase of our friendship so a new phase could begin. I have learned that the death lodge conversation is appropriate not just for the end of life; it is a wonderful way to stay current in relationships. I was having a conversation over lunch recently with someone who asked me how the work that I do with Zen Caregiving Project informs my relationships. I said I believed that most of the people in my life know how I feel about them, so there is very little unfinished business. I like to think that when I step away from an encounter with a friend or family member, they know that I forgive them, I welcome their forgiveness, I feel love for them, I appreciate them, and I know it is possible I will never see them again. This is how I want to live, making sure my relationships don't carry unresolved issues. I wish this for you not only in your caregiving but in all the relationships in your life.

It is likely that in the life review process unresolved issues in current and former relationships will come up. This is an opportunity to mention the practice of the death lodge, and to share the elements of the conversation with the person you are caring for. If the term *death lodge* is intimidating, you can call it something else or simply frame it as a way to attempt resolving any relationship issues. As already mentioned, you may be able to step in as a surrogate to help bring closure to past relationships when the person with whom there is unfinished business is not available.

Forgiveness?

Expressing each of the five death lodge statements authentically may be extremely difficult in some relationships. The person inviting a death lodge conversation may have suffered terribly because of the way they were treated, and they may not be able to forgive the person who hurt them. Getting to forgiveness can often be extremely tricky, and one's relationship to forgiveness is deeply personal and often complex. When someone resists expressing forgiveness, perhaps you can help them recognize that the behavior that causes pain to others is often the result of the perpetrator's unhealed emotional wounding. And that in recognizing the suffering of the person who harmed them, it may be possible to find compassion. From this place of compassion perhaps forgiveness for shortcomings can be expressed. One does not have to condone harmful behavior to express forgiveness.

Forgiveness is also an act of love, lifting a burden needlessly carried. If you can forgive someone, you move closer to fully opening your heart to them. Saying, "I love you" to someone who has harmed you conveys that you have loved life, the life that has for better or worse included them. It recognizes that the relationship has been part of who you are. When life as we've known it is ending, we see its preciousness, the way it has shaped us into who we are today. Even those who have hurt us represent an experience in a rich life that is ending. Saying goodbye to the life that is slipping by has a way of leading the person who is dying to a place of deep love and appreciation that includes everything and everyone.

I am not sure how you can love life and not feel boundless gratitude, even for the difficulties you have experienced. Saying "thank you" to someone who has caused you pain can be a recognition of the difficult lessons you have learned because of their unskillful behavior. Or it can convey gratitude for any positive aspect of the relationship.

The death lodge conversation is about setting down one's burdens, once and for all. Forgiveness, love, and gratitude feel much better than anger, hatred, and resentment. Who does not want to feel better at any stage of life? If not now, when? As a caregiver, you can use conversation to help the person you care for liberate themselves from whatever they are leaving behind, including unresolved issues in their relationships.

It is very likely that most of your time as a caregiver is filled with completing tasks that must get done. Adding deep conversation, which can take time, to your to-do list may not feel very realistic. Stay open and attentive to the right moment for you and the person you are caring for. Perhaps you can take a chance by putting off some task that needs your attention and raising a topic that has not been discussed. It is difficult to imagine that you will ever regret trying to engage the person you are caring for in a conversation about loss. The reward of such conversations is a feeling of intimate connection and the warm glow that comes from knowing you've provided a spacious, caring container to hold another person's most deeply held stories about their fleeting and precious life.

[Practice]

- Take some time to think about the losses experienced by the person you are caring for. Make a list of whatever comes to mind.
- Once you have a list, think about their willingness to talk about the losses associated with their illness. What have you noticed about their willingness to discuss difficult topics?
- Finally, think about what you might say or do to engage them in a conversation about loss.
    - What timing seems most appropriate for them?

  - How can you meet them where they are in terms of their openness to such conversations?
  - What specific questions might you pose that could lead to a meaningful conversation?
- If you are not comfortable inviting a conversation about loss with the person you care for, consider who else might be appropriate for such a conversation. Think about how you might approach this person to ask for their support.

CHAPTER 21

End-of-Life Wishes

Death is inevitable
Let us prepare together
Share with me your wishes
I will do my best to honor them

This chapter will support you to work with the person you are caring for to document end-of-life wishes in the form of an advance directive. You are encouraged to complete your own advance directive, if you have not already done so, and to consider what it would be like getting something other than what you want at the end of life.

When caring for a loved one or client, it is extremely useful to learn what they would like when they reach the end of their life. Most people don't want to think about their end-of-life experience. However, thinking about what a good death would look like and sharing those desires with a trusted family member or friend is more than worthwhile. This is especially true for people who live with chronic and serious illnesses and require ongoing care. I would like to share two stories that illustrate the relevance of knowing the end-of-life wishes of the person you are caring for.

Fulfilling a Wish Versus Making a Decision

Several years ago, a dear friend of mine received a phone call dreaded by anyone whose parents are still alive. Kathy learned that her father had suffered a serious stroke and had been rushed to the hospital. As soon as possible, she flew across the country to be with him. When Kathy and her sister arrived at the intensive care unit, they found their father unresponsive and on life support.

As the designated medical proxy for her father, Kathy had to decide how to proceed with his care. In conversations about his end-of-life wishes long before his stroke, Kathy's father had been very clear with her that he had no desire to be kept on life support if ever he could not live without it. Once she learned that his chances of recovery were remote at best, Kathy decided to remove her father from life support, thereby honoring his wishes. Kathy instructed the ICU team to remove her father from the machines to allow his natural death. Although it was painful to say goodbye to their father, Kathy and her sister did not have to bear the weight of such a difficult decision. The decision had been made for them by their father.

As I shared earlier, when my mother suddenly became gravely ill, she was eventually rushed to the hospital via ambulance. When I arrived to be with her the following day, I found my mother unresponsive in a bed in the ICU, being kept alive by machines. In the hours after my arrival, my father, sister, and I sat in my mother's hospital room in a state of disbelief, not knowing what would come next. The uncertainty we were feeling was the only positive thing we could hold onto. We clung to the possibility that she would eventually get well enough to have the ventilation tube keeping her alive removed. After a few long hours, the medical director of the ICU department came in to talk with us. He explained that given the range of comorbidities my mother had been living with for years, he saw very little possibility that she would recover to the point of breathing without intubation. If she did recover, it would take several months and intense physical therapy to get her breathing on her own again.

Since my mother was never willing to talk about what was important to her regarding her end-of-life care, we had to decide for her what was best in this situation. After the ICU physician left the room, the three of us discussed what to do. The doctor's assessment was difficult to absorb. I don't think my father, in his state of shock, really understood clearly what the doctor had conveyed about my mother's chances of survival.

I was the one to utter the horrible words that propelled us into the next phase of my mother's death. I explained that I felt the most compassionate decision we could make was to instruct the palliative care team to remove the life-support machinery once my brother and other family members could arrive. It was a painful decision that was left to us to make. We were not carrying out our mother's wishes; we were making the decision on her behalf. The distinction may seem subtle or even insignificant under such circumstances, but I think had we known what our mother wanted, it would have been easier for us to make the decision.

Conveying one's wishes for end-of-life care is a gift to those who will carry out those wishes. Being clear with loved ones about what is important and desired becomes part of the legacy that is left behind after death. If you do not know what the person you care for wants, it is important to ask. Even if you think you know what they want at the end of life, it is always worthwhile to revisit their hopes and expectations from time to time. As we age, attitudes about what matters at the end of life change and evolve. If you encounter resistance to discussing end-of-life wishes, you might try explaining that being clear about what is desired is a gift for those who will be making the difficult decisions. Pushing through resistance to discussing one's end-of-life wishes is an act of love and generosity.

Resources for Documenting End-of-Life Wishes

These days, countless resources are available to support conversations about wishes for end-of-life care. The most important part of the conversation about end-of-life wishes is designating a healthcare agent or proxy, the person responsible for advocating for the patient in the hospital environment. The proxy carries out the wishes of the person who is nearing the end of life. Not everyone is cut out for the role of proxy. It should be someone who will be comfortable carrying out wishes, even if they or others do not agree with those wishes. To be a strong advocate, the proxy must be able to push back against the pressures of a healthcare facility or family members who disagree with the wishes as documented on a healthcare directive form.

If you are in the role of primary family caregiver, you may have been asked or will be asked to be a healthcare proxy. It is vital that you consider whether or not you are the best person for the role. Sometimes, spouses are not the best candidates for proxy, given their emotional involvement. It really depends on the person.

Thankfully, we have reached a point where medical providers ask for a healthcare directive before performing certain procedures. It is hard to imagine that the person you are caring for has not been asked to complete a healthcare directive in which they have designated a healthcare decision-maker. Many healthcare directive forms are very basic. At the minimum, anyone dealing with a serious illness should have a Physician's Orders for Life-Sustaining Treatment (POLST) form signed and shared with a primary care physician and a loved one who can access it when needed. The POLST form does not replace an advance medical directive, although it does focus on four areas of decision making: (1) whether or not CPR is wanted, (2) the types of medical interventions that are desired, (3) under what circumstances artificially administered nutrition would be desired, and (4) designation of legally recognized decision-maker.

Other healthcare directives may include questions that invite consideration of a fuller range of serious illness and end-of-life scenarios. They will cover such topics as:

- What are your priorities or goals if you experience a serious healthcare issue?
- What does comfort care mean to you?
- How involved do you want to be in the decision-making about your care plan?

- What do you want your healthcare team to know about you?
- Whom do you want to spend time with when you are seriously ill or at the end of life?
- Where do you want to be if your health worsens?
- Under what circumstances do you want to be placed on life support?
- How do you want to be remembered?

In the resources section I offer a list of organizations providing materials you can use with the person you care for so they can record their wishes.

Your Own Advanced Medical Directive

I often ask caregivers who attend our courses whether they have completed an advanced medical directive. It is typical for about half the participants to respond that they have not. I always ask them, "What are you waiting for?" It is never too early to think about your priorities for when you are seriously ill or dying and to complete an advance directive. Life is unpredictable. We never know when tragedy may hit and prevent us from conveying our wishes for treatment.

If you are asking the person you care for to think about and record what they want when their illness worsens or when they reach the end of their life, it will be helpful if you have done the same already. If neither you nor the person you are caring for has a healthcare directive in place, perhaps you can approach it with the goal of completing them together. The activity of completing an advance directive can bring up strong emotions, and it is best to be ready for this.

An Advance Medical Directive Is No Guarantee

Engaging in conversations about end-of-life wishes can return a sense of agency to the person living with serious illness. Some people who arrived at the guest house had carefully documented what they wanted for their final weeks of life. It is easy to get attached to the idea of things working out exactly how you want them to. If someone is used to exerting a high degree of control in their life, they will likely want to control things as they are dying. This may work out for some people; however, it may also lead to disappointment or even anger at the end of life.

While it is vital to think about and share what you want at the end of your life, I believe the real work is preparing to not get what you want. I have shared with my wife that when I am dying, I want a view of a natural setting. I want windows open for fresh air, sunlight, and the sound of birds and wind in the trees. As my designated healthcare decision-maker, she knows exactly what I believe will contribute to a good dying experience. However, I also know that the things I desire at the end of my life may not be possible. It is impossible to know what we will encounter when the time comes.

Ultimately, I hope I can surrender to the dying experience, and I can only achieve that if I can accept my circumstances, no matter what unfolds. I can train my mind to prepare for this kind of radical acceptance in this moment, when I am healthy, by cultivating mindful awareness. In my many years of mindfulness practice, I have been learning to be with things just as they are, no matter the circumstances. It does not work to be with things as they are in one context but not in another. If calm and an open heart is to be achieved at the end of life, it is necessary to begin practicing mindfulness and compassion in the face of disappointments today.

A useful question to ask oneself when completing advanced medical directives is, "What is it like for me when I do not get what I want?" Or, "What will it be like for me if I do not get what I want at the end of life?" Although thinking about end-of-life wishes is extremely important, it should not create unrealistic expectations. When you imagine what you want for yourself at the end of life, it is best to acknowledge the very real possibility that you may not get those things. This does not have to mean that you will be denied calm and peace in the face of death. Do not wait to plan for your death or the death of the person you are caring for. Because one thing we know for certain is that death will come.

[Practice]

If you have not thought about your end-of-life wishes, I encourage you to consider the questions below. If you can, write your responses in a journal. Writing down your thoughts will make it easier for you to record them later in an advance directive document. Do not rush through these questions. If needed, set this activity aside, and return to it at another time. Share your responses with a trusted friend or family member.

If strong emotions arise for you as you consider these questions, practice allowing the emotions to move through, as you did in chapter 5.

- Who would you designate to make healthcare decisions on your behalf if you were unable to make decisions for yourself?
- If you were found unresponsive and in cardiac arrest, would you want cardiopulmonary resuscitation (CPR) performed to resuscitate you?
- If you were found unresponsive but not in cardiac arrest, would you want full treatment with the goal of prolonging life by all medically effective measures? (In addition to standard nonintensive medical care, this could include intubation, advanced airway interventions, medical ventilation, and cardioversion.)
- If you were found unresponsive but not in cardiac arrest, would you want medical treatment that avoids burdensome treatment? (This might include noninvasive positive airway pressure, IV antibiotics, IV fluids, and comfort care measures.)
- If you were found unresponsive but not in cardiac arrest, would you want comfort care measures only? (This treatment might include medication to relieve pain and suffering, use of oxygen, suctioning, and manual clearing of airway obstructions.)

- If you could no longer take in food by mouth, would you want artificially administered nutrition (e.g., a feeding tube)?
  - If you would want artificially administered nutrition, for how long?
- If you had a serious life-threatening illness,
  - How much medical treatment would you want to prolong your life?
  - Where would you want to be as your situation worsens?
  - How open would you like to be with friends and family about your situation?
- Which is a priority for you, prolonging your life or improving the quality of your remaining life?
- Whom would you like with you as your illness progresses and death gets closer?
  - Is there anyone you do not wish to see when you are seriously ill or getting nearer to death?
- How do you want visitors to behave toward you?
- Do you have any favorite music you would like to hear when you are resting?
- If you were confined to a bed, what would make you feel comfortable?
- What other comfort measures might you want when you are seriously ill or dying?

CHAPTER 22

Preparing for the Dying Phase

As the final moments of your life slip past
The preciousness of each breath is brought into clear focus
May I view each moment as a treasure
The memories of which I will cherish forever

This chapter invites you to consider what is likely difficult to think about: the dying experience of the person you are caring for. The information offered here will help you make the dying experience of that person as gentle as possible.

"Love is watching someone die." This moving line from a favorite song of mine sums up what it has been like for me being with people who are actively dying. Beneath the pain and disorientation, there is always love. As a family caregiver, watching your loved one die will likely be the most difficult thing you ever have to do. And it is probably the last thing you want to spend time thinking about. However, since your care will likely include the final days and hours of life of the person you are caring for, preparing for their death is a worthy activity.

I will assume your motivation to provide the best care possible for your loved one includes being there for their dying experience. This chapter is intended to support you in making your loved one's transition to death as easeful as possible. As you know, ideally, that work begins long before the person you are caring for nears the end of their life.

When it becomes clear that the person you care for is entering their dying phase, it may be helpful for you to step back and get perspective on your role as a caregiver. This reevaluation may need to happen amid a storm of strong emotions. Even if you have been caring for someone for many years and have watched their illness progress, a terminal prognosis will likely cause emotional distress, including sadness and fear. As part of reevaluating your role, you might ask yourself, "What is my intention in this experience? Or, "How can I offer the best support possible until the moment of death?"

Based on what the person you are caring for has previously shared about their end-of-life wishes, you will want to consider if anything different needs to happen now that death is within sight. It may be time to ask if the person you are caring for wants anything specific from you as they move toward death. At the same time, you will need to be realistic about what you can and cannot provide during this time. You may need to accept that it will be impossible for you to ensure that they get exactly the death they want.

Planning for the Unknowable

The dying experience is unpredictable. It is impossible to know how the time leading up to death will unfold. During this uncertain time, everything you have learned and practiced about cultivating mindful awareness becomes especially important. As the end of life approaches, every moment shared with the person you are caring for gains profound significance. How attentive can you be to each moment as it passes, never to return again? Despite the sadness, this final phase of life can be a time of wonder and deep connection. It can be a very healing time for the person who is dying and for those around them.

In the final days of life, you will not be able to anticipate what will happen next. I learned from Frank Ostaseski that it helps to surrender to the not-knowing. Describing his own experience of the uncertainty of accompanying someone who is dying, Frank shared, "I move from one moment to the next new moment, without an idea of where the process is going." All you really need to know is what is happening in this very moment. Staying with each moment of the experience without needing to know what will happen next requires an ease with uncertainty and a deep, abiding trust in the dying process.

Depending on your relationship to the person you are caring for, your grief may prevent you from providing reliable care in the face of increased emotional and physical burdens. So even though you have been a primary caregiver up until this point, you may find that once the person you are caring for begins to die, you are too emotionally distressed to provide the care that is now needed. Or you may want to spend this precious time being with the person you are caring for without needing to tend to all the tasks related to their care.

Calling In Additional Support

Once it is determined that the person you are caring for is terminal, and that their death is in the foreseeable future, it is time to line up the support you will need to best address their new set of needs. The effort required in tending to a person who is nearing death should not be underestimated. Nearing the end of life, the person you care for will sleep more, which under normal circumstances would provide you with some relief, but if they are a close friend or family member, you will likely want to be with them even as they sleep. Sitting with a loved one who is dying is a potent time. Once they enter the active dying phase, you will ideally have others present to support you with your own physical and emotional needs. Understandably, when a loved one is dying, many family members have difficulty leaving the bedside to address their own basic needs.

Whether or not people have shown up in the past to assist you with caregiving, it is likely that they will recognize the importance of stepping up during the final stage of life of the person you are caring for. Many people find it difficult to know what to offer when someone is dying. It is really helpful to let people know clearly what you need to feel supported.

As the person you care for gets closer to death, they will lose the energy required to engage with visitors. The dying person may not be able to accommodate the desires of the people who have waited until now to visit and say goodbye. It may even become necessary for someone to turn visitors away. Even close family members will eventually be left on the outside as the dying person goes inward and no longer has the strength to interact with others. It does not matter how bonded the dying person has been to a partner, family, or friends; eventually, they will stop communicating with others during the active dying process.

By making the right decisions early, you will have the support of trained professionals in advance of the end-of-life phase. Thankfully, our health system is designed to provide additional care for people living with a terminal condition in the form of palliative care and hospice care. It is never too early to begin asking about these forms of care so you and the person you care for are prepared to make the transition to comfort measures.

Palliative Care

Sadly, many people living with a serious illness experience a lot of unnecessary suffering. The practice of palliative care, as the word *palliate* implies, was developed to minimize suffering. Although palliative care is often viewed as something for those at the very end of their life, it can make a huge difference in the life of someone living with a serious illness who may be several months away from their death. If your loved one is living with a serious illness, palliative care can do a lot to improve the quality of their life and the lives of those around them.

Palliative care is relatively new in the United States, having become a recognized medical school subspecialty in 2006. In the period between 2000 and 2020, the percentage of hospitals in the US with palliative-care programs increased from 24.5 percent to 83.4 percent. Despite this steady increase, many people who would benefit from palliative care services do not receive it. One of the reasons is the widespread assumption that palliative care is only relevant in the context of end-of-life care.

My friend Tom Almeida, who cofounded the Infinito conference and network to increase awareness of palliative care in his home country of Brazil, has a wonderful way of describing palliative care for those who may not be familiar with it. He uses the metaphor of air travel. Imagine you are traveling in coach class to a destination you have spent years planning to visit. Midway through the flight, the pilot announces that there will be turbulence ahead. You are told the flight will get very uncomfortable and your destination may even be changed due to the disruption. However, a flight attendant informs you that even though things are about to change, you are being upgraded to first class. The service you receive will address all your needs. The flight attendants cannot prevent the turbulence, and they don't know where you will end up, but they will be there to make your time onboard as comfortable as possible. You will have the support you need during the rough flight.

As a caregiver, you are making the trip with the person you are caring for. Like the service provided by the flight attendants in this imaginary scenario, the support a palliative care team provides will be beneficial for you as well as the person you care for. Typically, the team will include physicians, nurses, nurse aides, social workers, chaplains, nutritionists, physical and occupational therapists, a care coordinator, and even volunteers. Each team member will be focused on minimizing the suffering of the person you are caring for and others in their support network. The palliative-care team will address the symptoms of illness; however, addressing the cause of disease will be left to other departments. That is to say, the patient can continue to see a specialist, whether it is an oncologist, neurologist, pulmonologist, nephrologist, and so on. The continuation of curative care is a normal part of palliative care, but once someone is admitted into hospice, medical interventions intended to cure disease are discontinued. In hospice, comfort measures are prioritized.

Timing of Hospice

I have recently been supporting my friend Susan, who is caring for her mother who was diagnosed a few months ago with a terminal illness. Susan's mother is a fighter, determined to do whatever she can to halt the progression of her cancer. Susan has tried to engage her mother in conversations about end-of-life wishes, but her mother has resisted acknowledging the terminal nature of her illness. After a few weeks of chemotherapy took its toll on her quality of life, Susan's mother began to accept that she would likely not recover from the cancer.

A notable part of their recent conversations has been the topic of when to enroll in hospice. Like many people, Susan's mother had a lot of confusion about what palliative care and hospice are and what it means to enroll with a hospice agency. Susan's mother assumed that enrolling in hospice was only relevant if her death was imminent. This is not the case, as Susan informed her.

It depends on the type of illness, but in many cases, enrolling in hospice will prolong the life of a patient with a terminal diagnosis. Hospice is focused on maintaining and improving quality of life. Palliative care, which is part of hospice care, is focused on alleviating suffering. Many patients do not realize that enrolling in hospice allows them to receive the supplies and treatment that will make living with a life-limiting illness much easier, even if they are months away from dying. Typically, patients are eligible for hospice for a duration of six months, but it is very common for patients who outlive the six-month limit to be recertified and enrolled again.

Although some residential hospice facilities exist, most hospice care is delivered in-home, whereby members of a care team visit the patient's home. The care team is composed of the following types of caregivers: volunteers, nurse aides, social workers, chaplains, registered nurses, and physicians, all of whom will make home visits.

The first day of enrollment in hospice care can be overwhelming. A nurse or social worker will come to the home and conduct an intake interview. If the patient can advocate for themselves, they will be asked if they are requesting hospice enrollment. It needs to be the patient's decision, unless they are incapable of making their own healthcare decisions. The intake interview will be followed by visits by the other caregivers assigned to the patient. The process can be exhausting for someone with low energy.

On day one, the patient should also be ready for the delivery of disposable and durable medical supplies. The arrival of items like pain medications, disposable briefs, bed pads, wound dressings, plastic basins, a wheelchair, an oxygen machine, and maybe even a hospital bed may feel shocking to someone who does not currently need these items. Such items can be an alarming sign of things to come for someone who has not thought much about the changes their body will go through as death gets closer.

Once the decision to enroll in hospice has been made, I strongly suggest sharing with the person you are caring for what to expect on the day of the intake process. You can explain why it is helpful to have the items and people in place, even though it is possible they will not be needed any time soon. I have seen how distressing it can be when someone who needs pain meds or oxygen has to wait for a prescription order to be delivered because it was not on site in advance.

While it is common to hear about how kind and supportive in-home hospice caregivers are, they are only human. I have also heard stories of frustration that hospice caregivers have been slow to arrive when a family member needs support. In-home hospice is not the same as being in a care facility. A dying person's condition can change quickly. Pain can break through the current dosage of pain medications, and unexpected symptoms can appear suddenly. The patient might experience confusion or extreme anxiety. Family members should have a plan in place to support each other while they wait for a hospice agency caregiver to show up when needed. This is simply a reality of high patient caseloads and other conditions that sometimes make an immediate response impossible.

Staying calm in the face of a crisis can be extremely difficult, yet it may be exactly what is needed. Panic never really helps; it only agitates everyone involved and disrupts clear thinking. A perceived crisis is precisely when you should return part of your attention to your breath to disrupt thoughts that may be triggering panic, an expression of the amygdala hijack explained in chapter 13.

I encourage you to discuss with the person you are caring for what kind of crisis would warrant a call for an emergency medical response. Once enrolled in hospice, ideally you will avoid calling 911. By enrolling in in-home hospice, the person you are caring for has decided they want to remain at home for the dying experience. Being rushed to the hospital increases the likelihood that they will stay there until their death. I have great respect for the people who work on emergency medical teams and in hospital emergency departments. And I have also heard many stories about nonresuscitation orders being disregarded when 911 is called.

Hospice as Threshold

Enrollment in hospice is a threshold, a clear indication to a person with a terminal illness and their community that it is time to prepare for the end of life. Even if the person you care for stays in hospice for many months, the threshold of enrollment offers an opportunity to begin saying goodbye. If steps have not already been taken, it could be time to begin the death lodge process covered in chapter 20. You can support the person you are caring for in the process of saying goodbye to friends and family.

I recall Frank Ostaseski saying, "Dying is a spiritual experience and not a medical emergency." Humans have always cared for their dying. Only relatively recently have we ceded care of the dying to hospitals and medical professionals. You have everything you need to be a companion to the person you are caring for as they transition into the dying phase of their life. Although the input and support of medical professionals is of course beneficial in providing relief from physical discomforts, you have an essential role to play in the final weeks, days, and hours of life. You do not need to be anything other than who you are to provide emotional and spiritual support as someone dies.

Limitations on What You Can Change

The first thing to remember is that while you may be able to affect subtle changes in the dying experience, there are limitations on what you can change. You may be able to make the person you are caring for more comfortable, but you will reach a point where there is nothing more you can do to support them. A lifetime of causes and conditions have led up to the dying experience. It will be too late to change certain patterns of behavior or thinking that are having a negative impact on the dying experience.

I have learned more from my wonderful teacher Eric Poché about how to show up for someone who is dying than I've learned from anyone else I have worked with over the years. Eric was the volunteer program manager for Zen Hospice Project for much of its history. I had the privilege of serving with Eric for about fifteen years before he retired. When any concern or judgment would come up about how someone's dying experience was going, Eric used to say to us, "This person is simply having the dying experience that they are having," and he would go on to say that it was not for us to change it. By the time someone is dying, there has been too much that we simply haven't had control over. This holds true even when the person we are caring for is a family member. As much as we may want to ensure they experience what we would consider a "good death," it is foolish to project our own wishes onto someone who is dying.

Dying Time Is Sacred Time

The closer one moves toward death, the concerns that previously occupied their thoughts become less relevant. Even patients who have tried to orchestrate every aspect of their illness and care must eventually let go of their need for control. It simply becomes too exhausting, and priorities shift. Concerns shift from the practical to what I would describe as the spiritual. Even if someone remains conscious far into their dying process, they will likely become very quiet and contemplative.

The time of active dying is sacred. To honor the dying experience,

I recommend removing as many of the signs of a medical condition as possible. Even though the person dying may not be very aware of their surroundings as they begin to actively die, the environment will leave a lasting impression on you and others who are present.

I believe it is an act of kindness to minimize sounds, light, and other external stimuli that may disturb whatever internal process the dying person is experiencing. Try to keep lights low, and avoid loud conversation and unnecessary noises. Ask yourself what kind of conditions in the space around you would make you feel at peace if you were in the bed dying.

It is possible that the person you are caring for will ask in advance for physical contact as they approach death, like hand-holding or caressing. If you are told this in advance, then you are following their wishes. However, if you are not fulfilling the dying person's expressed wishes, you might ask yourself if you are touching them to address your own emotional needs or because you think it is bringing them comfort. I believe that once someone begins to actively die, physical touch may disrupt their process of shedding their body.

I remember a very moving encounter with the adult daughter of a woman who was dying at our hospice house. The daughter took a break from her mother's bedside to sit on the back deck of the house. I could hear her crying, and I went to join her. I quietly sat down beside her and after a moment, she said, "I know it is now too late."

"What is too late?" I asked.

"I know it is no longer okay to touch my mother, since she is already crossing over," the daughter replied.

The sensitivity of the daughter to her mother's process was deeply moving. It confirmed something that I too had sensed in dying people. They reach a point in the process when touch is no longer supportive. This does not mean you mustn't make physical contact with the person you are caring for as they die, only that you should pay very close attention to what you are seeing and what you think they need. Their needs should always take precedence.

If you are present when death comes, I encourage you to take your time. There will be a stillness like nothing you have known before. I believe it continues to be supportive to the person who has just taken their final breath if you and others can sit quietly and let things settle. Take in the fullness of the moment. It might be very helpful for your grief process to watch the subtle changes of the body as it cools and becomes something other than the person who just died.

Reading this, it may be impossible for you to imagine the moment of death of the person you are caring for. You do not need to. Let yourself move into the experience one breath at a time. The death you witness will likely be as painful for you as it is mysterious. It will be a moment forever etched into your memory.

[Practice]

Take a moment to settle your mind by focusing on your breath. Then think of the person you are caring for and how you want to show up for them in their dying experience. If big emotions arise for you, practice noticing where the emotions are showing up in your body. Do your best to stay with the question, "How do I want to show up for _______ as they are dying?" Or, "What is my intention for _______'s dying experience?"

In your journal or on a piece of paper, write a succinct intention for the kind of support you want to provide to the person you are caring for as they die. Keep this intention someplace where you will be able to find it again. Revisit your intention from time to time as you learn more about the end-of-life wishes of the person you are caring for.

CHAPTER 23

Rituals to Mark Loss and Death

With all beings throughout time
I will honor loss and grief
By giving myself to the moment
Making a ceremony of this passage

Recent studies have provided proof of what humans have always known, that rituals, simple or complex, are extremely useful in processing grief. This chapter offers guidance for creating your own rituals to mark loss and death.

Throughout history, humans have metabolized loss through the enactment of ritual and ceremony. The internal process of coping with major life changes has always found its way to outward expression and release through action that links what is personal to the sacred or universal. Engaging in ritual, we tap into a field of energy beyond what is contained in the body and mind. Ritual offers a reminder that we are part of something boundless and timeless, a sacred container that holds our narrow experience of loss. Connecting to the universal provides a new and necessary lens through which we can see our loss as both essentially human and as an expression of the divine.

A growing body of psychological research shows that the use of ritual promotes healthy grief processing. Perhaps most importantly, the research finds that rituals return a sense of control to a situation that feels beyond our influence. Rituals also allow those who grieve an opportunity to acknowledge the reality of a death or loss while providing a tangible outlet for the thoughts and feelings associated with the loss.

Whatever your spiritual or religious background, you likely have engaged in rituals that are prescribed to mark significant life events, including loss. Rituals performed in the context of religious tradition connect the mourner to the larger body of adherents, past and present. Every religion and culture has established rituals to honor the grief experience as well as some type of funeral or memorial ceremony. Meanwhile, it is also possible for mourners to create their own rituals. I invite you to embrace the concept of "self-generated ceremony" to mark and honor your experience of loss. Self-generated ceremony provides a spacious container for mourners to create their own rituals based on what has personal meaning for the life event being marked.

Following the death of my mother, I decided to go off to the desert and fast for four days and nights. I chose a cave I had previously used for shelter during a ritual fast. It was situated on the slope of a mountain ridge overlooking a wide-open valley. My intention for the fast dedicated to my mother was to work on shifting my relationship to her by letting go of the living, embodied mother and calling in the spirit mother I could still feel connected to, but in a new and different way.

A daily ritual I engaged in during my solo time was to eat a small amount of food in the morning, even though I was technically fasting. My mother often expressed concern that I was too thin and did not eat enough. Ritualizing the simple act of eating a small portion of dried fruit, nuts, and hot broth seemed a fitting way to honor my mother and the love and support she extended to me. I received each precious bite of food as a gift, thanking her and assuring her that I would take care of myself, just as she would want.

It was impossible for me not to also acknowledge the generosity of the great earth mother, the source of the food I was taking into my hungry body. In the process of extending gratitude for the life-sustaining nourishment, my birth mother became entwined with the earth mother. There was no separation between my birth mother and the earth mother; they were one. This was exactly in line with my intention. I view my mother now as inseparable from the maternal energy that gives birth to everything and holds each of us as we journey through life. That is where my mother has gone, and that is the spirit energy to which I can connect daily.

My solo time entailed other rituals to mark my passage into a new phase of life. My days were filled with conversations with my mother, reflection, screaming, crying, laughing, meditating, and intention-setting. When I completed my time in ceremony, I descended the rocky ridge, returning to camp to share my story and then a few days later returning home to resume my life there. I arrived home feeling much lighter and as though I no longer carried the heavy burden of my grief. It was as if I had left it in the desert, in a place that will forever be associated with that experience of deep ceremony.

If the story of my grief ritual strikes you as peculiar, that is a reflection of the beauty of self-generated ceremony. What feels meaningful and useful to me may not be meaningful and useful to others. What works for you may not work for me. I appreciate the permission that self-generated ceremony bestows on each of us to carefully consider what we need from ritual and to craft it for ourselves.

I was very fortunate to have been able to break away for several days to enact my grief ritual. However, it is also possible to create rituals that take very little time. Do not underestimate the impact of less elaborate and shorter rituals. You might find a simple gesture or ritual that you enact daily for a period of time. I encourage you to work with whatever resources and with however much time you have. A ritual devoted to processing loss can be as simple as a daily prayer, a walk, or dedicating a meal to the deceased or to whatever is no longer in your life.

Creating Your Own Grief Ritual

In my experience of creating meaningful grief rituals for myself and others, I have identified three key elements that can be used as a template when creating your own. I label these elements *story*, *surrender*, and *succession.* Although I explain the template in terms of the ultimate loss, that of a death, it can be used when processing the grief that arises following any type of loss.

Story, the first phase of a grief ritual, is a celebration of who or what has been lost. It is the full acknowledgment of your relationship with the source of your grief, a chance to look back on how things were before the death of a loved one. The possible activities associated with this element of the grief ritual are storytelling, dispersing the possessions of the deceased, displaying or reviewing the creations of the deceased, or even releasing anger or regret regarding the deceased. It is an opportunity to review the role of the deceased in your life up until now.

Surrender is the in-between transition phase of the ritual. In this phase you let yourself acknowledge whatever emotions arise for you as you steep yourself in the fullness of your loss. This is a moment to be with the unrestrained expression of your grief. In this phase, you will be best served by staying in contact with your present-moment experience. This phase might take the form of a meditation, a silent reflection, final words of goodbye to the deceased, a prayer, tears, or even wailing. In this phase, you are releasing your grief emotions.

Finally, in the *succession* phase you are planting seeds for what comes next in your life. Recognizing that so much is different now, this phase is future oriented, helping you to reimagine a new way of being. Succession supports you in finding purpose in the loss. It invites you to consider the legacy left by the loved one who has died and how you might support and spread that legacy. You might contemplate whether you will do anything differently in the future to honor that life that has passed. Other activities associated with this phase could be sharing out loud an intention or finding an object that represents what you learned from the deceased.

Integrating Objects into Ritual

Whatever form your grief ritual takes, you might find integrating certain symbols or objects extremely supportive. For instance, holding an object during part of your ritual and then releasing it can help you let go of painful memories, missed opportunities, or difficult emotions. Objects can include photos, articles of clothing, favorite books, jewelry — whatever feels meaningful to you. For my mother's funeral, my father, siblings, and I each wore a piece of her jewelry. The brooch I wore during the funeral went out to the desert with me, and I used it in the ritual I described earlier. It currently sits on an altar in my home, reminding me of my mother. Salt was commonly used in rituals we offered to family members mourning the death of a loved one who died at our guest house hospice facility. Family members would hold a pinch or two of salt in their hand while recalling their loved one out loud. Then they would disperse the salt into a tall vessel of water and watch as it dissolved. The salt was still present in the water but no longer visible. I am also fond of using rocks in grief rituals as a talking piece to hold while sharing a story. They can be held during rituals and then returned to an outdoor space to symbolize something or someone you are letting go of. Or they can be placed in a pocket or purse or set on a shelf and kept as a reminder of some new intention or commitment to yourself. As part of your ritual, objects can be buried, submerged in water, burned, or placed in a special location in your home.

Embodying Ritual

Some types of movement can be extremely powerful in releasing stuck energy in the body. I have found dance to be an effective way of processing grief when I cannot otherwise release it. Many people are self-conscious about dancing while in groups, and if this is the case for you, try to find a place where you will have privacy. You might dedicate a period of movement to celebrating the body that is still sustaining you. Free-form movement and dance are wonderful self-care practices for releasing tension or processing emotions.

Music or sound can be extremely evocative in grief rituals. You might incorporate a song that was a favorite of your deceased loved one, which may help release stuck emotions. Or you might go to a place where you know you will hear the sounds of birds, flowing water, the wind, rustling leaves. These sounds can be calming and can help you feel connected to the natural, enduring world that holds your experience of loss.

If the weight of your grief prevents you from crafting something elaborate, you might enact something very simple like a walk dedicated to the person you are grieving, as discussed above. On the way out, let yourself think of the person, recalling your relationship and what you learned from them. When you are ready to return, you might pause for a few moments to let go of any thoughts and check in with any emotions that are present. On your return walk, think about ways you can honor the person by carrying forward their legacy or sharing what you have learned from them with others.

Whatever you plan for your grief ritual, it can be helpful to let go of any attachment to it going according to your plan. If you are not familiar with enacting rituals, it may feel awkward or forced. This is natural. Try to push through any resistance, and trust in the power of the ceremony, regardless of how it unfolds. Though the impacts of a grief ritual may be subtle, you may still experience a sense of release or lightness. Trust that your body and psyche will remember the enactment of ritual.

Sharing Rituals with Others

You might consider inviting family and friends to participate in a grief ritual. Others can play a part in crafting a ritual, or you can invite them to participate in a ritual you have crafted to meet your own needs. Enacting rituals with others can enhance its effects since you have witnesses who effectively hold the story of the ritual with you. The collective enactment of ritual also supports you to feel connected to a community of mourners and thus less alone in your grief.

Most people will find comfort in the ceremony a funeral or memorial provides. Every religion and spiritual tradition has its communal rituals of honoring death and supporting the grief process, rituals such as the wake in Catholicism, *shiva* in Judaism, or *terahvin* in Hinduism, to name just a few. However, you are not limited to these more traditional and communal forms of marking death. If your grief is heavy and debilitating, you may choose to ask a trusted friend to organize a separate ritual. However, while a more elaborate ritual experience crafted by a friend will likely be impactful, don't let it replace simple rituals you can integrate into your life on your own.

Divine Nature of Grief

Although difficult and exhausting, the period of intense grief following a death of a loved one is sacred time. Profound loss can disrupt life like nothing we've known before. When we are at our most vulnerable, we are also closest to the divine, though that may be impossible to appreciate when we are in the depths of grief. When we occupy this holy space, every action takes on the poignancy of a ceremony, fostering deep meaning in our life. When we look back on times of intense grief, they take on a kind of preciousness. Even the difficult times become closely associated with the loved one no longer present.

My sister and I were in charge of cleaning out my mother's closet a few weeks after she died. My mother loved shopping for clothes and held on to everything she ever acquired. Sorting through her things with my sister took on the quality of ritual. Each article of clothing that passed through my hands felt at once precious and insignificant. Old memories would arise and trigger strong emotions. My sister and I talked at length about our mother, and there were extended moments of silence as we filled and labeled black plastic bags for donating to the resale shop. Though it would have been easy to put off the task, my father was ready to let go of this powerful reminder of my mother's presence in their home. We were each taking steps to move into the next phase of life without her. As painful as that time was, I knew the pain was necessary and that it would not always be like that. Rituals, elaborate or simple, serve as a reminder that we can trust the process of grief without knowing where it will lead us or how long it will take to get to wherever it is taking us.

[Practice]

Take a few moments to recall a past loss. It could be the death of someone close to you, or it could be the end of a relationship or a phase of your life that came to an end to make way for something new. As you think about a past loss, without judgment, notice if any grief arises for you.

Think about how you could honor your grief or the memory of a person through the enactment of a simple ritual. If it is helpful, try using the *story, surrender, and succession* template to craft your ritual. You can ask yourself, "Is this a ritual for me alone?" "Do I want to include any friends or family members?" "Where would I like to enact this ritual?" "What objects or elements would be suitable for my ritual?"

If there are constraints on your time, I would not worry about when you will carry out the ritual you've imagined. Thinking about the kind of ritual that would support your experience of loss will prepare you for when you do have the time to enact the rituals that you create for yourself and others.

INTIMACY

Enlightenment is intimacy with all things.

— Dogen

We want to attune ourselves carefully to our body and mind so that we can feel it when we are out of line with our deepest intention. We want to cultivate that intimate knowing without words and ideas, that intimacy with our self, so that we can tell if we are living our life the way we really want to.

— Zenkei Blanche Hartman

CHAPTER 24

Maintaining Healthy Boundaries

I am a relational being
Who needs others in my life
And I have the right to protect myself
From difficult encounters

This chapter will help you understand the dynamics of boundary issues and how to cultivate greater awareness of when your emotional boundaries are crossed. You will also learn useful ways of responding when someone encroaches on those boundaries.

Many caregivers I meet talk about their difficulty with maintaining healthy emotional boundaries. A common thread is the question of how to best respond when someone says or does something that causes a caregiver distress. Boundary issues are often related to others' expectation that a caregiver do more or accept more than what is comfortable or reasonable. Even when another's behavior or words activate big emotions and you feel a need to protect yourself, it is possible to respond with skill and in a way that strengthens the relationship.

What Are Emotional Boundaries?

Boundary intrusions occur when someone oversteps the limits of another's comfort zone. They are common in the caregiving experience because they are common in life. Interacting with others regularly means that we will bump up against each other's emotional boundaries. There is really no way around it.

If we think of our body and mind as part of a collective field of energy and matter, then there are no boundaries between us and others. You could say, in an absolute sense, there is no separation between us and others. Yet, in more conventional thinking, we exist in a world that requires the boundaries our minds create. And while we know suffering is simply part of life and to be expected, when our emotions get triggered because of another's words or actions, we shouldn't pretend it isn't happening or that it is necessary to put up with it. You have the right to protect yourself from difficult encounters. The key is being aware enough to choose a response that does not worsen an already stressful situation or dismiss the importance of your health and well-being. It is possible to respond to challenging boundary situations and maintain a sense of agency and well-being.

Here are some examples of boundary issues:

- An adult daughter caring for her father feels a boundary is crossed when he asks her to clean his house so he does not have to pay a housekeeper.
- A brother feels a boundary is crossed when his caregiver sister won't let him speak for himself during a medical appointment.
- A nurse feels a patient has crossed a boundary when the patient asks for their personal phone number to call after work hours.
- A spouse of someone living with dementia feels a boundary is crossed when they are accused of trying to cause pain while assisting the spouse with bathing.

In our Mindful Caregiving Education courses, we help people understand the dynamics of boundary issues and how to cultivate greater awareness of when they are happening. Having a framework to understand this relational dynamic can be very empowering for times when you feel something is wrong but do not have an effective way to address the source of your discomfort.

Fluidity of Emotional Boundaries

Our emotional boundaries are constantly shifting. Whether or not you feel an emotional boundary has been crossed can depend on how well-resourced you are feeling on any particular day. Sleep, nutrition, relationships, and stress can all influence how we experience others' behaviors. Emotional boundaries are fluid, changing from day-to-day, even moment-to-moment.

It is helpful to remember that not only will your own boundaries get crossed, but you may cross others' emotional boundaries. When you cultivate self-awareness you both prepare for someone crossing your emotional boundaries and you also more readily see when you are about to cross someone else's boundaries. As a caregiver, if you are not paying attention, you will cross others' boundaries. Recognizing boundary issues and learning healthy ways of coping with them is vital to the long-term well-being of both caregiver and care recipient.

Using Mindful Awareness as a Guide

Mindfulness is a key tool in recognizing and working with boundary issues. Sometimes you may not realize that your boundaries have been violated; you just feel that something is wrong. When you lack clarity about a situation, it is easy to react unskillfully and make things worse. Since you can use mindfulness to slow down and deepen your awareness of emotions and physical sensations, you can also use it to guide your response to boundary incursions. The body does not lie; it will send signals that something is not right, even before you understand what is really happening. Learning to attune to physical sensations is the first step in navigating the tricky terrain of emotional boundaries.

Paying attention to the body through mindful awareness can also help you pause before reacting unskillfully. A favorite piece of wisdom, attributed to the writer/philosopher Viktor Frankl is, "Between stimulus and response there is a space. In that space is our power to choose a response. In our response lies our growth and freedom." When you pay attention to your body and mind, you can choose your response in any given situation. You can respond to boundary issues in a way that clarifies your own needs while conveying clearly that the relationship matters to you.

Applying STOP to Boundary Violations

An excellent tool to use when another person's words or behavior do not feel comfortable is the STOP practice you learned in chapter 8. As soon as something doesn't feel right, simply *Stop* what you are doing. Return your attention to the body by *Taking a breath* or two. Then *Observe* the situation. Finally, once you have a better understanding of what is happening and you feel stabilized in your body, you can *Proceed* in a skillful way that addresses the boundary incursion causing you distress.

You can think of an emotional reaction to what someone says or does as an alarm going off, telling you something is not right. Such signals should not be ignored or pushed aside. Avoiding boundary issues may work in the short term, but it is not sustainable. Over time such denial takes a toll, resulting in resentment and stress, and ultimately contributes to burnout. While the internal process of following STOP will not put an end to boundary intrusions, it will very likely return a sense of control to you when you feel helpless in a situation. You may be familiar with the old saying "If you can't change your circumstances, change your attitude." The STOP approach helps you shift your attitude. It changes your internal emotional experience and supports a skillful outward directed response to boundary incursions. Let's look more closely at each of the steps of the STOP practice when used in the context of boundary challenges.

Stop

It may not always be possible to literally stop what you are doing. Stopping really means shifting your attention and noticing your internal response to the circumstances you encounter. Stopping is the action you take to initiate each of the following steps; it is your starting point.

Take a Breath

When you pause to follow an in-breath and an out-breath, you are returning to your awareness of physical sensations, which are immediate. While it is helpful to focus on the breath, in this step you can also attune to other physical sensations, such as feeling your feet on the ground or the points of contact between your body and the chair you are sitting on. You could also shake out your hands or place a hand on your chest over your heart. When observing physical sensations, you shift into direct experience. You are in the moment. There is no past or future when it comes to observing physical sensations. It is when we begin to layer stories or thoughts onto sensations that we leave present-moment awareness.

Focusing on physical sensations also disrupts the thought process that may be triggering big emotions. As explained in chapter 5, disrupting such thoughts will help lessen the duration of a challenging emotion. Present-moment awareness is the best way to support a response that is free from distraction or emotional agitation.

Observe

With this third step of the STOP process, it can be useful to label your emotions and identify where they are showing up in the body. Most importantly, you can ask yourself, "What exactly is upsetting me?" You might also consider, "Is something other than what was said or done contributing to the feeling that my emotional boundaries have been crossed? Am I feeling well-rested? Has an earlier encounter lingered with me? Have I had enough to eat or drink today? What is the context for the boundary incursion?"

One inquiry I find extremely useful when dealing with boundary issues comes from a communication process known as nonviolent communication, founded by Marshall Rosenberg. The inquiry invites you to consider what lies behind the behavior that crossed your emotional boundary. In other words, what unmet emotional need activates the person's behavior? Such consideration in no way absolves the person who crossed your boundary of accountability for their actions, but it may generate a more compassionate response and inform the way you advocate for yourself. For example, someone who yells at their caregiver spouse for going out for coffee with friends may be feeling lonely or isolated. Or perhaps they are fearful of what could happen when left alone.

Proceed

The final step in the STOP approach when used with boundary challenges is to decide and initiate what comes next. This response can be immediate, or it could unfold over a longer period of time. Sometimes the most skillful response to a boundary violation is to separate yourself from the person who crossed your boundary so you can collect yourself and spend more time in the *Observe* stage or on deciding how best to proceed. I realize this is not always possible. If you cannot get away, the pause and reflection that STOP provides will still help you respond in a way that does not make matters worse.

Maintaining Agency

Choosing a response represents the agency you can maintain even in uncomfortable circumstances. Although nothing can eliminate boundary intrusions, you can maintain a sense of freedom in how you respond. For a caregiver who is feeling trapped in their circumstances, this can mean a lot.

Though it may feel natural for the caregiver in the example above to react by yelling back at the spouse to defend their decision to take a break from caregiving, choosing a more skillful response will usually diffuse the situation. The caregiver could say that they will ask someone to come stay in the house while they are away or suggest a plan of action if something were to go wrong. In other words, you are doing or saying something that addresses the underlying needs driving the triggering behavior.

Conveying a clear boundary to a loved one or to someone you

are caring for can be an act of compassion. It conveys that you are committed to caregiving while also being committed to taking care of yourself. These commitments are not separate. Finding ways to advocate for yourself will support better caregiving since you will feel you have more control over your own short-term and long-term well-being.

Even when you respond skillfully to boundary intrusions, your response may not always be received well. It is important to accept that you cannot control someone else's response to your clarity regarding emotional boundaries. You could say that the way the other receives your clarity is up to them. It is their business.

Responding Skillfully in the Context of Dementia

Addressing boundary issues when caring for a loved one living with a dementia-related illness will require some very different tools. It is likely that your skillful outward response will not change the behavior that crosses your emotional boundaries. However, using STOP to be less reactive in a boundary situation may support you to feel better about yourself. In such situations, this approach supports your sense of calm and presence. In my experience caring for people living with dementia, although words may not have an impact on behavior, a calm attentive presence often does help diffuse difficult interactions.

Your Feelings Are Valid

Resentment, anger, or despair are each natural feelings that you may experience in the face of ongoing boundary incursions by the person you are caring for. When you experience these emotions, remember to practice self-compassion. Let yourself be human, with all the vulnerability and fallibility that being human entails. Even though you may try to be skillful in the face of ongoing boundary intrusions, at some point you will likely do or say the wrong thing. When you react unskillfully, do your best to forgive yourself, and move on. Next time you may do better. And then you may slip up once again. Navigating boundary issues is simply part of caregiving. All you can do is keep working to maintain healthy boundaries to support both your relationship to the person you care for and your long-term emotional health.

[Practice]

Stop. Take a breath. Observe. Proceed.

Using the STOP practice in your imagination is great training for making STOP a conditioned response to boundary situations. After practicing a few times, try using the STOP out in the world. Before long, it will be automatic. Eventually, you won't even need to think about the four steps, since they will all just happen naturally.

- Find a quiet and comfortable place.
- Close your eyes, and let your attention rest on two or three breaths.
- Now think about a recent boundary intrusion you experienced, remembering as many details as possible. Notice if you have an emotional response to the memory.
- Imagine yourself applying the STOP practice in the midst of this boundary intrusion.
    - Imagine what each step would feel like for you.
- Would you proceed differently if you could do things over?
- Notice if any self-judgment comes up for you, and if so, let go of judging thoughts.

Following this contemplation, take some time to record in your caregiving journal what you noticed about applying the STOP practice.

CHAPTER 25

Working with Storied Self and Essential Self

Celebrating the beauty of silence
And the gift of words
May I have wisdom and courage
To discern which is most useful

This chapter introduces two aspects of self, essential and storied, and ways to apply one or the other, depending on the circumstances. Shifting from one aspect to another is how you use the self therapeutically in your caregiving.

Years ago, while I was sitting with Nancy, a resident on the palliative care ward at the city hospital, her family members arrived for a visit. Nancy's daughter was accompanied by her two teenage children. As Nancy's daughter approached the table where we were sitting, she said, "Hi, Mom! It is great to see you! I brought Jenny and Lisa with me." Nancy was living with Alzheimer's disease, and I could see that the approach of these three visitors with their excited energy agitated her. As her two granddaughters expressed their greetings, Nancy took on a confused look. Her daughter saw this and said, "You remember me, Mom, don't you? It is me, Susie. I was here last week." As Susie took a seat at the table, Nancy looked at her and then in turn looked at each of the granddaughters. She did not seem to register who they were. After a moment of tense quiet, Nancy gently patted the table with both hands and said something about the dinner she was waiting for. At that point I left, leaving Nancy to visit with her family.

The encounter was painful to witness. It seemed Nancy was in distress, as was her daughter. It was as if Nancy knew she should remember but clearly did not. Nancy's daughter seemed desperate to have her mother remember who she was. I have seen this dynamic many times. Understandably, it is extremely difficult for family members to accept that they are not recognized by a loved one living with a dementia-related illness. I think if I had asked Susie at the time what she wanted most for her mother, she would probably rank Nancy's comfort and happiness above remembering that she was Susie's mother. However, Susie's apparent desire to have her mother remember her did nothing for Nancy's comfort and happiness. In fact, it seemed to make Nancy feel bad.

Perhaps you have experienced a situation like this with a family member or friend. You want to help them remember who you are. Perhaps you have even told them stories about shared experiences to prompt their memory. When someone begins to lose their memory, it impacts family and friends by robbing them of the person who holds the other end of the very important thread of relationship. Looking for ways to help them remember may feel like support for the person with dementia, but ultimately the inclination is probably more about your needs than theirs.

When I think back on situations like the one just described, I am struck by the irony that letting go of the story of our relationship to someone living with dementia can actually allow for a deeper feeling of connection and ease. If we can meet the person living with dementia in the moment with pure presence, they will likely feel more comfortable being with us, less alone, and ultimately, happier. Sadly, the alternative is to set them up for failure, frustration, and confusion.

Thinking about *how you are showing up* in the caregiving relationship is essential to the quality of care you provide, regardless of the diagnosis of the person you are caring for. In other words, it helps to consider how you express who you are when you care for others — and to consider how you express the "self" in your caregiving.

The Self as Caregiver

You may be wondering what I mean when I use the word *self.* Defining *self* is complex since it can be explored from several different perspectives — psychological, spiritual, scientific, and philosophical, to name a few. How you think about self depends on how you think about who you are and on how you think others perceive you. For the purpose of looking at the use of self to enhance caregiving, I define *self* as how you show up in the world, or simply how you answer the question, "Who am I?"

Essential Self

In part 1, we looked at ways of reaching a state of pure presence. When we are fully present to what is happening right here, right now, we experience what Buddhist teachings refer to as "no-self." This is another way of saying that we drop the story of who we are and experience a state of timeless, boundless consciousness. This may sound complicated, but it is actually the simplest and most straightforward thing we can do as human beings. Many names have been used to describe this state of being, such as *essential self, authentic self, big mind, true nature, soul,* and *transcendent self.* I am fond of the term *essential self,* so this is the term I will use.

Our essential self is an expression of who we are that has nothing to do with our past conditioning, our stories, our tastes, our preferences, our political leanings, how we look, and how we think about others. This state has nothing to do with how we want to be perceived by others, or even how we see ourselves in the world. This aspect of self is only attainable when we are in a quiet, attentive state of nondual awareness, where we experience our oneness with all phenomena. When interacting with others, our essential self is expressed as our full presence to the moment and to the person we are with. This expression of essential self can play a vital role in caregiving under particular circumstances, which we will explore below.

Storied Self

Most of the time, we show up for caregiving and for the relationships that fill our lives with our "storied self." The storied self can be called *ego*, *persona*, *self-concept*, *self-image*, or *personality*. This expression of self is characterized by the story we tell others about who we are. It is our desire to control the circumstances we encounter, and it conveys our expectations for how others should show up in relationship to us. Storied self is our unique expression of how to be human. For most of us, it is our default way of expressing who we are in the world. This aspect of self becomes fixed in our minds, even though each of us is actually changing all the time. Storied self is necessary for functioning in the world, and we could not accomplish much without it.

Your Two Aspects of Self

Take a moment to think about how you would describe your storied self. How would you introduce yourself to someone you were meeting for the first time if they expressed curiosity about you? You would probably not have any difficulty listing the elements of who you are. What roles do you play? Whom do you like to hang out with? What activities do you enjoy? What objects are meaningful to you? What are your favorite foods? Where did you grow up? Storied self is the default expression of self.

Describing your essential self is, on the other hand, quite difficult. It can be very challenging to even talk about. I would say essential self is almost ineffable, or beyond words. We can talk around it, but it can be difficult to touch it with words. Like storied self, the expression of essential self plays a different but equally important role in caregiving.

Both these aspects of self are worthy, and looking at certain scenarios will further clarify how each aspect of self can enhance your caregiving.

When you start integrating mindfulness into caregiving, you learn to shift from the storied self to the essential self. In this chapter we are exploring ways of shifting between the two aspects of self, depending on what is most supportive to the person you are caring for.

Leading with Storied Self

Connecting with others through the expression of storied self is one of the great joys of life. Sharing memories, naming what is important to you, and expressing curiosity about the person you are caring for supports connection and a sense of community. Most of the time, leading with storied self is the most natural way to deepen a caregiving relationship. Below are some situations when showing up with storied self is most supportive.

Caring for the Homebound

I know from my own experience of being ill that when you are confined to a bed or even to your home, your world can start to feel really small. Someone experiencing prolonged illness may long for news of the outside world or may want to live vicariously through others' experiences. When encountering this situation, it can be very useful to share stories of your own encounters out in the world or to engage the person you are caring for in recalling fond memories of times when they were healthy and independent. The person you are caring for may crave a story to distract them from the monotony of their limited activities. When we share stories, we are expressing storied self.

Supporting a Life Review

As we touched on in our discussions of loss, most people approaching the end of their life will engage in the process known as life review. The storytelling part of a life review is a perfect example of engaging the storied self. Nearly everyone I have met at this stage expresses a deep need to share the significant experiences of their lives. Before they can loosen their attachment to the past, the person experiencing a terminal illness needs to share their stories. If you observe someone moving into this stage of the dying process, showing up with the storied self is extremely supportive. In this process, you as a caregiver can be supportive by eliciting stories and helping someone remember and celebrate who they have been. Sometimes, eliciting life review stories means telling the person who is dying what they have meant to you, and they may need your help remembering certain experiences.

Engaging with Clinicians

The most skillful clinicians are able to see their patients as whole people. They view patients as more than just folks displaying the symptoms of a particular illness. Taking the time to understand the patient's history, the clinician gains insights into all that has led up to the current circumstances. Learning about a patient's prior lifestyle helps overcome latent biases and offers direction for determining a unique and impactful care plan. It is necessary to share stories if you want the clinician treating your loved one to see them as more than just a manifestation of symptoms, so it requires the expression of storied self. In your role as family caregiver, you may be able to fill in some of the blanks left by the person you are caring for when they are seeing a medical practitioner. This requires that you lead with your storied self in sharing the patient's story and your relationship to them.

Using Humor

The basic human need to experience levity and humor exists even when someone is living with a chronic or serious illness. As a caregiver, please do not overlook the importance of helping the person you care for access lighthearted humor. Recalling humorous events or pointing out the irony or absurdity of certain situations is a valuable gift you can bring. Humor is born of one's ability to view a story or situation differently from what is obvious. Shifting perspective to see something as humorous requires leading with your storied self.

Leading with Essential Self

Shifting to essential self is not always easy; however, it offers numerous benefits and thus is useful to practice. Expressing essential self is another way of integrating mindful awareness into your caregiving relationship. Below are some situations that are best addressed by expressing your essential self.

Caring for Someone with Dementia

In our example above, had Nancy's daughter Susie approached her with quiet focused attention, it is very likely that Nancy would not have experienced uneasiness. By leading with her essential self, Susie could have created safety for her mother. Susie's essential self would not have needed Nancy to be anything other than who or how she was in that moment. When we express essential self, we convey an acceptance of everything as it is. Marguerite Manteau-Rao, author of *Caring for a Loved One with Dementia*, points out, "The essential self is what allows us to relate to the person with dementia, particularly in the most advanced stages when the person's constructed self has eroded the most." Essential self has no attachment to controlling things or having them be different and in this way can reduce suffering. By expressing essential self to someone living with dementia, we meet them where they are rather than expecting them to meet us where we are.

I have learned over the years that people living with dementia remain very attuned to the emotional energy of the people around them. Approaching them with a calm presence supports them to feel more at ease with their circumstances, even though they may be confused about who you are. If the person you care for is more at ease, they may be able to access memories that otherwise would remain outside their grasp. Even if they cannot, they will still benefit from your presence rather than be made to feel like they are doing something wrong.

Authentically expressing essential self with someone who has forgotten who you are can be extremely difficult if you are a family caregiver. It is a painful experience not to be recognized by a loved one who is losing their memory. Difficulty accessing essential self with a loved one is understandable. If it is not possible for you, please be kind to yourself and remember to express self-compassion.

Accompanying Those Nearing Death

When a loved one is approaching death, it is best to minimize any chaos or agitation in their space. A quiet, responsive companion following the lead of the one who is dying is most supportive. Apart from soft expressions of love, there is really no need for a lot of words. In the final days and hours of life, the one who is dying enters sacred space. In these final moments essential self won't disrupt their process. As difficult as it may be, it is most helpful to set your emotional needs aside and to let the dying person's process unfold however it does. At this point, you really cannot influence their experience, so it is best to let it be what it is.

When Someone Is in Denial

Many people facing a new diagnosis use denial as a coping mechanism. When a person is in denial, they have not yet acknowledged their acceptance of their current circumstances. This does not necessarily mean that they don't know what is happening but rather that they may not be ready to let others know that they know. Some people may need more time to catch up with the new reality. They may need more time to create and get used to a new story or self-concept.

If you are caring for someone who in your opinion is expressing denial, it really won't help to refute their position. It is best to wait until they are ready to acknowledge things for how they truly are. In this situation, it is skillful to express your essential self. This allows you to be a listening and caring presence without refuting or feeding their denial. The quiet presence of essential self conveys that what is true in the present moment is safe and does not need to be resisted. This safety and nonresistance includes your own emotions that may arise. Emotions can be just as they are without reactivity and without resisting or feeding them; they become part of what is unfolding in the present moment. Your essential self offers an invitation to join you in the truth of what is here and now.

When Someone Laments Lost Abilities

Many people with serious illnesses understandably express sadness over the loss of past abilities or freedom. I have often felt that they express their sadness to convey something about who they were so that I can see them more fully. In the chapters about loss, you learned ways of supporting others as they lose important elements of their self-identity. When someone laments the loss of past abilities or freedom, you can convey that what is here in this moment is more than enough, that they are not in any way "less than." Essential self has nothing to do with one's past abilities or activities. You will be most supportive by expressing essential self and inviting the one you are caring for to meet you there with their essential self. With essential self, nothing is missing; everything is included. This takes the form of your quiet, openhearted presence that is ready to receive any story and hold it.

I hope by now you see the difference between storied self and essential self. Moving between the two will not always be easy. An ability to discern which aspect of self is most useful, and your ability to pivot between the two, will enhance your caregiving. The more you practice mindfulness through meditation or by sustaining focused attention on a task, the easier it will be to become a therapeutic presence to the person benefiting from your care. As you deem appropriate, do your best to apply each aspect of self when providing care. See what you notice.

[Practice]

- When you next engage with the person you care for, pause for a moment to consider whether your storied self or your essential self will be most supportive in the interaction. There is no right or wrong selection; just notice and experiment.

- After your encounter, see if you can identify which self was prominent. Ask yourself what might have been different had you led with the other aspect of your self.
- Note which aspect of self feels more comfortable or natural, and why.

CHAPTER 26

Sharing Your Story

When unexpressed, heavy are the burdens I carry
Sharing my story lightens my load
May I find the courage to express what I hold
in this caring heart

This chapter highlights a core need among caregivers to be witnessed in their story of caregiving. Ways to establish a safe container for storytelling are introduced, including helpful guidelines for storytelling.

Human beings are storytelling creatures. It is simply what we do. We are at our best when we find time to listen deeply and share authentically. Our stories, when expressed out loud, breathe life into our internal world. Even a young child, with the most basic of language skills, expresses excitement and urgency when given the opportunity to tell their story. The need to share stories with others continues throughout life.

Hearing yourself tell a story is nourishment for the soul. This type of nourishment sustains you for whatever comes next. The attention and deep listening of others encourage you to explore different ways of looking at your circumstances. By telling your stories, even when they are about struggle, you have the opportunity to observe yourself and your actions. Stepping back and hearing yourself share, you naturally consider how you might approach your life differently. This type of processing is part of emotional growth.

Held stories need to be processed, and we give them the attention they deserve by telling others what we have experienced. We need to know that our life matters. Sharing how you feel about your life gives meaning to the activities and events that fill your days. Part of the harm of social isolation is the absence of a witness. If you do not share your story, it is easy to become stuck in old patterns of behavior and thought. And this absence of an outlet for your stories is a form of suffering. French philosopher Gaston Bachelard put it this way: "What is the source of our first suffering? It lies in the fact that we hesitated to speak...it was born in the moments when we accumulated silent things within us."

In earlier chapters, I shared why it is important for the person receiving your care to share the story of their illness or to engage in a life review. It is also beneficial for you to share your stories of caregiving with a friend or someone other than the person you are caring for. Storytelling not only gives you an opportunity to look at how you are meeting your caregiving responsibilities, but it also minimizes the sense of isolation that so many caregivers experience.

It is possible that as a caregiver, you feel you don't have time to share with others what it is like to be a caregiver. However, sharing your stories with others is a worthwhile use of whatever free time you have. If you encounter a lot of difficulty in your caregiving, sharing your struggles with others will help lift the burden of negative emotions you may be holding about the experience. Not having an outlet to share what makes you feel anger, frustration, sadness, resentment, or other negative emotions makes caregiving painful, and sharing your story provides a release for such emotions.

Take a moment to ask yourself, "Who are the people in my life who will truly listen to my story? Is there someone I trust to listen without expressing judgment or challenging me? Who is willing to give me their undivided attention?"

Establishing Ground Rules for Sharing

Even if there are people whom you trust and who are happy to spend time listening, it may be useful to establish some agreements before sharing your story. Our world is filled with distractions. It can be difficult to create the conditions that allow you to tell your story without being interrupted or ignored. The devices we carry with us are an endless source of distraction. And, of course, the demands of caregiving may make it difficult to share a story without interruption.

You may need to have a "conversation about the conversation" with whomever you plan to share your story. Give yourself permission to ask for what you need to feel safe and truly witnessed. Before asking a friend or family member to listen to your story, you might ask yourself some questions: "How can I convey my expectations for sharing my story? How much time am I asking for? Do I need whoever is going to hear my story to put their phone into silent mode? What kind of place will feel comfortable for me to share openly? Will I ask the person who receives my story to share a story of their own? Do I need to ask for an assurance of confidentiality?" Your answers will help you establish the conditions supportive to sharing your story.

Perhaps you are thinking that this all sounds pretty complicated; however, establishing a safe container is important. Otherwise, you might be telling your story when the person who is listening becomes distracted by a phone call, a text, or a news flash, or they run into someone who wants to say hello. These sorts of interruptions can be very unsettling when you are sharing the intimate details of something you have dealt with while caregiving.

If you are unable or choose not to establish the conditions you need to feel safe in sharing a story, I caution you not to give away your story too quickly. In other words, test the waters. You might share a story superficially and see if the person or people you are sharing it with are attentive, receptive, and curious to hear more. If they are, then go into more detail or allow the emotions associated with the story to arise. Sharing a story superficially is not quite as satisfying as sharing it in detail, but it may be more satisfying than not sharing it at all.

Guidelines for Storytelling

Gigi Coyle and Jack Zimmerman established what they call the "intentions of council," which they shared in their book *The Way of Council.* I find these intentions extremely helpful for establishing the conditions that support authenticity and vulnerability when sharing a story. The intentions are *spontaneity, being of lean expression, listening from the heart,* and *speaking from the heart.* You might introduce these guidelines in your conversation about the conversation.

Spontaneity means you trust that what needs to be witnessed will emerge as part of your story. There is no need to prepare in advance what you are going to say. Try to accept that the story that emerges when you have the opportunity to share it is exactly the story that needs witnessing. If you are with more than one other person who will also be sharing their story, being spontaneous means you are not preparing what you will share while another person is telling their story.

"Being of lean expression" means recognizing that not every detail can be covered in your storytelling. Trying to remember the details so you get your story just right can be a big distraction. Your story does not have to be the perfect telling of what happened. Share what feels most essential to you. It feels really good to be witnessed, but don't take advantage of others' time and attention if you want them to listen to you again in the future. Being of lean expression means you also honor the amount of time that has been agreed on with the one hearing your story.

Listening from the heart or listening generously is really about paying careful attention to the person sharing a story. You can make the person speaking the object of your focused awareness, just as you would focus on your breath or other physical sensations in meditation. If there is an agreement that all people present are sharing a story, you can model the kind of listening you would like to receive from others.

Speaking from the heart involves recognizing the value of expressing your emotions as a relevant and important part of your story. In other words, can you share the emotions that arise as you are telling the story or the emotions you had when you were experiencing the situation you are speaking about? In terms of storytelling as a way of supporting your emotional well-being, it may be more beneficial to share the emotions associated with the situation than the details of what happened. Do your best to be kind to yourself as you share your story.

Finally, I recommend that you get agreement from whoever is listening to your story that they will keep it confidential. This will support you in sharing the more intimate details of your story. And of course, only share these kinds of details with those you really trust.

I have been using these intentions for many years and have found that when agreed on, they create enough safety for storytellers to go wherever they need to in their sharing. You may be willing to take a chance on sharing your story even when your expectations are not met. It may take a few attempts before you find the ideal person, group, or setting to share your story. Profound sweetness and satisfaction come from sharing honestly and deeply under the right conditions. This is worth working for and, if necessary, waiting for.

When There Is No One to Turn To

You may feel like you no longer have someone with whom you can share your story. This is fairly common for people who have spent years as caregivers. If this is the case, there are still ways for you to talk about your caregiving experience. Numerous organizations support caregivers by offering support circles, both in person and online. Some of these organizations are listed in the resources section at the back of this book. If you have not done so already, you might begin by checking with the health system the person you are caring for is part of.

If you know other caregivers, you could invite them to meet and share stories about their experiences. I often hear from caregivers that it is helpful to hear from others who are dealing with similar situations. If not in person, you may be able to find an online forum to connect with other caregivers. If you are able to coordinate a group, I highly recommend that you introduce the guidelines shared above. By doing so, you create a safe container for you and others to share openly. These intentions also ensure that everyone knows that the kind of sharing and listening you are inviting is different from daily conversations. In fact, while you might leave time at the end for open conversation, it is helpful to agree on how much time each person has to share. A timekeeper can notify each speaker when their time is up.

Many Ways to Tell Your Story

If you do not have an opportunity to share your story out loud with someone else or with a group, you could record your story in a journal. The writer and Zen practitioner Natalie Goldberg celebrates the worthiness of writing down our stories. In her seminal book *Writing Down the Bones* she writes, "We are important and our lives are important, magnificent really, and their details are worthy to be recorded. This is how writers must think, this is how we must sit down with pen in hand. We were here; we are human beings; this is how we lived." I believe this sentiment also applies to sharing stories orally. Your story is worthy of sharing with others.

By expressing your story either out loud or in writing, you will more readily make meaning of your circumstances. Gaining some perspective on mistakes, difficulties, or conflicts helps build resilience. The perspective you gain by witnessing your own story allows you to come up with different explanations about what happened and why. When you tell a story, you free yourself from being stuck in your interpretation of an experience. Attachment to the story can be a source of suffering. When you speak about an experience, you not only loosen the hold of emotions associated with the story, but you may discover new approaches to dealing with similar situations in the future.

When sharing your story of caregiving out loud or in writing, try not to limit yourself in how you tell it. There are many ways to tell a story. Although you may have an attentive listener, you are not telling the story for entertainment value. You may end up entertaining the listener — making them laugh or keeping them on the edge of their seat with anticipation — but that need not be the purpose.

Your storytelling style may be to share what happened sequentially, in the order it happened. However, it is just as worthwhile to jump around in the narrative. You may find it helpful to reenact what happened with movement or gestures. You may choose to read something you wrote. You may need extended periods of silence to remember something or to settle yourself. You decide how to tell your story so that when you finish, you feel fully witnessed.

When Fear Shows Up

A lot of fear or anxiety can arise when sharing a story from a place of vulnerability, especially if more than one other person is listening to you. For years, when it was my turn to share in storytelling councils, my body would tremble. This was my body expressing my fear of judgment as well as my excitement about what I was sharing. The uncontrollable trembling was extremely unpleasant, and I did my best to hide it, until I realized trying to hide it just made it worse. I discovered it only went away once I acknowledged it out loud, making it part of my story.

Some fear is natural if you are not used to sharing how you feel with others or talking about situations where you think you could have done better. It might be helpful to invite fear in as what is true for you in the moment. Do your best to keep it from getting in the way of telling your story. You could try telling whomever you are talking with that you feel a bit unsettled. You could also invite a few moments of silence to focus on your breath as a settling meditation. And then, as you have practiced in earlier chapters, let part of your attention be on where the fear shows up in your body, and just keep going with the story that needs to be shared and witnessed.

Guiding Questions

When you do not have one particular story to share, it is still beneficial to talk about your experience as a caregiver. Whether you are talking with one other person or a group, it may be helpful to have a few guiding questions to shape what you will share. Some questions that can help guide you are:

- What challenges do you experience as a caregiver?
- What joys do you experience as a caregiver?
- What are two or three strengths you bring to your caregiving?
- Is there anything you would like to improve or change in your caregiving?
- What have you learned about caregiving?
- What do you wish you had known about caregiving when you were first starting out?
- What would you like new caregivers to know about the role?
- What do you notice about your experience listening to others in a group setting?

There are no right or wrong answers to these questions. Your honest responses are what matters most. Hearing yourself address one or more of these questions will allow you to assess how you are doing in your role as a caregiver, not in terms of success or failure, but in terms of tracking your well-being.

Sharing your story not only supports your emotional health and well-being, but it also benefits the listener. Whether the person you share your story with has been a caregiver, is currently a caregiver, or will someday be a caregiver, hearing your perspective on the role can help them gain insights on what it means to offer care to another person. If the people you share your story with can relax into listening, they too will experience a deep sense of connection and intimacy. And you will be giving them permission to share their story when they need to.

[Practice]

Is there anything about your caregiving experience you would like to share with someone you trust? This could be an experience of doubt or overwhelm or a mistake you made. It could be some disagreement you had with the person receiving your care. It could be something you have learned from your experience of being a caregiver. Or perhaps you recently had an experience of joy or delight while caregiving.

Think of someone who would be receptive to hearing your story. Reach out to this person and ask if they would be willing to give you some time to share a story about your caregiving. It would be helpful to be clear about how much time you are hoping to have with them. Or you could ask how much time they have available to be with you so you know what to expect. You could also let them know what kind of feedback, if any, you hope to receive in response to your story. Be ready in case the person you reach out to cannot offer you the time you need. Is there someone else you can reach out to?

If you do not have anyone you feel comfortable telling your story to, consider writing your story in a journal or even recording it as a voice memo on your phone. This too may allow you to experience the benefits of sharing your story.

CHAPTER 27

Healing Touch

When offering care
Let my energy bring calm and comfort
May these hands become tools for healing

This chapter introduces ways to bring more awareness to the simple act of physical contact with the person you are caring for. We will look at touch in the context of both practical assistance and companionship.

Much of what I know about offering touch to people living with serious illness I've learned from a dear friend and brilliant healer, Irene Smith. This chapter is inspired by and dedicated to Irene, who died in 2021. Irene devoted her adult life to offering and teaching touch awareness through a program she called Everflowing.

I first encountered Irene and her teachings in 1997, when I trained to become a caregiver volunteer. Until her death, Irene presented at nearly every volunteer training at Zen Hospice Project, since its inception in the late 1980s. When I first met Irene, as in every other training, she began her session in silence. She quietly took her seat and proceeded to rest her loving attention, in turn, on each trainee. She would hold a gaze for a moment or two and then move on to the next person. During this quiet ritual, the room remained absolutely still. This practice of hers was unsettling for those not used to such silent, noncontact intimacy. To me, it always felt as though she was seeing the truth of what was held in the heart of the person her gaze fell on. She was teaching us the first lesson of touch awareness.

Touch begins the moment you enter the space of the person you are caring for. Before any words are expressed or physical contact is made, we touch another with our eyes and our energy. People living with illness are especially sensitive to the energy around them and to the energy of those they interact with. Your calm demeanor, your eye contact, and your soft and steady voice convey essential information. Irene described healing touch as the application of mindful awareness to the touch relationship. Entering a room calmly and attentively, you invite the person you care for to trust your presence and to join you in deep connection. Even before physical contact is made, your steady energy will be felt as healing.

Touch Can Be Complicated for Some

Irene was extremely skillful in establishing a safe space for people to acknowledge and talk about past touch experiences that may have been dysfunctional or unhealthy. A history of unhealthy touch relationships can complicate care that involves touch. Irene would remind us that touch is the first language humans learn as infants. We are born with more than 4 million touch receptors in our skin. Each fingertip alone has about three thousand receptors. As newborns, we begin to understand our environment and the people in it through touch. As we grow, messages received from our family and society at large begin to shape the way we relate to others through touch.

Depending on your background, the thought of physical contact may evoke feelings of shame, arousal, embarrassment, inadequacy, or fear. Yet when the intention is to establish connection and to bring comfort to the person you are caring for, touch becomes an essential and sacred part of caregiving. The first step to pushing through any negative associations with touch is to recognize what gets in the way.

Once recognizing what makes physical contact difficult, you can begin to shift your relationship to healing touch. Proceed slowly, pay careful attention, and honor your boundaries. Try to trust that your resistance can shift over time. If your history of touch includes physical or psychological trauma, you may want to seek the support of a trained therapist to overcome resistance or discomfort.

The Need for Physical Contact Is Lifelong

The need for physical contact is obvious for the healthy development of infants and small children, yet the need for touch continues throughout our life. The physician Clifford Singer writes, "There is strong evidence that many older adults feel isolated, and that loneliness is associated with poor health and higher rates of mortality." Social isolation is common among the elderly, especially after the death of a friend, partner, or spouse. The lack of physical touch compounds the negative effects of living alone.

Since my mother's death, my father has lived on his own. He has made clear his desire to continue living for as long as possible in the home he once shared with my mother. My siblings and I talk regularly on the phone with my father, yet I do not get to visit with him as often as I would like. When I am there, I try to make physical contact as much as feels comfortable for both of us. When visiting, I ask my father for an embrace daily and try to place a hand casually on his shoulder or back as I move around him throughout the day. Like many older people who are inactive, my father has poor circulation and fluid accumulation in his lower legs. In addition to being red, the skin on his legs is often dry. I have used the dry skin on his legs, which he cannot easily reach, as a reason to apply lotion and engage in healing touch. I am fortunate that I was raised in a home where physical contact was quite natural, so this kind of contact is not uncomfortable for us. I use this time for conversation, making sure I keep part of my attention on the contact between my hands and his legs.

Benefits of Receiving Healing Touch

Even when there are others in the home, living with an illness can be very isolating. If you share a home with the person you are caring for, and the only physical contact you share with them lacks your awareness, they will likely feel a sense of isolation. When you offer touch with attention and sensitivity, the person you care for has an opportunity to feel their connection to the community and world around them. Healing touch also instills a sense of safety, not only with you as their caregiver but also with their own body that is in pain or not functioning the way it once did. Attentive touch can help put someone who is ill back in contact with their body after they have cut their awareness off from it due to constant pain and discomfort.

If the person you are caring for has lost their ability to verbally express themselves, touch offers an alternative way to communicate. Mindful awareness enables you to pick up on subtle physical cues that will help you understand how your touch is being received. I have sat at the bedside of people who were nonverbal and received useful information about what they wanted or needed by feeling the tightening or relaxing of their grip on my hand. Also, seeing someone's body tense up or relax can convey useful information.

It is possible that you have not given much thought to how you use touch when engaging in tasks that involve hands-on care. It is natural for even a loving spouse, partner, parent, or child to engage in daily caregiving tasks in a perfunctory or efficient manner. However, even when you are busy, tasks such as assisting with bathing, changing clothes, applying lotion, transferring from bed to a chair, and going on a walk are all opportunities to engage in healing touch. If you do not bring awareness to how you offer touch during these types of activities, the person you care for may feel unseen or like they are an object. Without awareness, physical contact can feel cold and mechanical.

Reciprocity of Healing Touch

Touch that entails careful attention and gentleness is healthy both for the recipient and for the caregiver. When physical contact is made through healing touch, the person you are caring for will experience the release of oxytocin, sometimes referred to as the "happy hormone." The release of oxytocin promotes positive feelings. Oxytocin is released even when we give ourselves gentle touch. It is an act of kindness to place a hand on your chest over your heart during a self-compassion break, since this kind of self-touch is comforting, even in the midst of a difficult situation.

Irene would often talk about the importance of self-touch, or "petting" as she would call it, especially for older isolated adults. She shared how she would take her time applying lotion to her arms and legs each day to make sure she experienced healing touch. I remember talking to Irene during the pandemic when she was living on her own and very isolated. She assured me that she was still engaging in her daily practice of applying lotion to her body mindfully.

Slowing Down and Paying Attention

As a caregiver, you can play an important role in modeling healing touch to those around you. Friends or family members who visit may be at a loss as to how they can be supportive, and you may be able to guide them toward gentle touch. Or you could encourage them to slow down and pay attention when engaging in tasks that involve physical touch. When observing an agency caregiver rushing through care because of their need to get to the next client or patient, you may be able to skillfully and gently suggest that they take more care with your loved one. This can be tricky, but if you do so with respect and compassion, you can remind them of the importance of slowing down and connecting through touch.

Slowing down and focusing your attention during activities that entail touch will enhance your sensitivity. In China and other Asian countries, it is common for people who are blind or visually impaired to work as massage therapists. Their limited ability to see does not prevent them from offering healing touch. In fact, their vision impairment makes them more sensitive to the places in the body where even subtle tension is held. I have noticed that when I am offering healing touch with gentle massage, closing my eyes actually helps me slow down and focus on the points of contact between my hands and the body of the person I am touching. It allows me to notice more about the person I am touching. This technique is also very relaxing.

Whenever your caregiver role entails physical contact, you have the opportunity to offer healing touch. It does not ask anything of you other than openhearted awareness. Through healing touch, you become the kind of healer the person you are caring for will benefit from. Becoming a healer, you allow your caregiving to be elevated from necessary action to an expression of loving-kindness.

[Practice]

I recommend this practice to help you relax before going to bed at night. All you will need is some type of skin lotion. Once you have your lotion and you are in a comfortable place, begin by closing your eyes and settling your mind for a few moments. Use your breath or physical sensations to interrupt any persistent thoughts that arise, just as you have practiced in earlier chapters.

Next, apply some lotion to your feet or lower legs. As you apply the lotion, you might consider how hard these parts of your body work throughout the day. Gently massage the lotion into your feet or legs, focusing all your attention on the sensations of your hands and the parts of your body that are receiving your touch. Give yourself over to the enjoyment of kind, gentle touch.

Spend as much time as you can, but at least five minutes. When you decide to end, pause and notice any sensations in your hands or in the parts of your body that received your touch. Notice what you feel in your heart and what thoughts are arising for you. If the experience was enjoyable, try to stay with the positive feelings for as long as possible. If judgment arises, do your best to return to sensations.

CHAPTER 28

Feeding Gratitude

When pain and suffering cast darkness
May I look more closely for the light
The bright warmth of gratitude is never far
I need only gaze upon it

In this chapter, you will be reminded that gratitude is always close. Even in the midst of difficulty, turning your attention to what is worthy of your gratitude can help you shift from stress or despair to well-being.

Gratitude is a salve for the burdened mind and the aching heart. When we are busy rushing around, trying to meet the demands of life, or when we are struggling with some challenge, our outlook can become narrow. If we stop to observe the mind in such times, we will notice that we have been in a very contracted state. In such a mind state, we see less. Life becomes very limited, and we can feel as though we are stuck in hardship where not much is possible.

If, in moments of stress or struggle, you can stop and consider what in your life is worthy of gratitude, you will shift into a more expansive mindset. The source of your stress or difficulties may not be eliminated; however, you will have more creativity, ease, and energy in dealing with the situation. Possibilities open up. Turning your attention toward what is good in your life feeds gratitude. As you build a habit of turning toward what you have to be thankful for, you strengthen a healthy mind state supported by gratitude.

Present-Moment Awareness Supports Gratitude

When you are in a contracted mind state and your focus is limited, it is difficult to remember to turn toward gratitude. However, as you strengthen your mindfulness practice, it becomes easier and more natural to pause in the midst of difficulty. Zen Buddhist priest and author Zenju Earthlyn Manuel acknowledges, "It is difficult to say thank you in the midst of the struggle.... If there is a long enough pause, many of us experience profound insight that we can use for the rest of our lives. And in that, we are more grateful for life, whether it is up or down."

When in a state of mindful awareness, you establish the conditions that support gratitude, and accessing it becomes quite easy. As you know by now, mindful awareness is about noticing what is true in the moment. In a state of mindful awareness, there is no room for thinking about what is missing or what could be better. Thinking about what is missing takes you out of the moment. When you pay attention to what is here and now, you see the abundance that exists in each moment.

In this moment, you have breath. You have your senses. Even if you have health issues, and aches and pains, you have a body that has sustained you and continues to do so. Your mind and memory may not be what they once were, but you have awareness. There is the blue sky above and the clouds, the sun, and the moon. There are trees, plants, and flowers. There is a roof over your head. You have life! Present-moment awareness will open up to appreciating the simple pleasures that you may overlook as you fulfill the demands of caregiving. Then, if you are blessed to have a family and friends and healthy food and comforts, there is even more that is worthy of your gratitude.

Of course, you have problems and difficulties like me and everyone else. Naturally, your mind will turn toward what feels challenging or what is missing. However, you also have a choice in this moment to stay focused on what you have. Focusing on what you have rather than on what is missing or what is problematic naturally evokes gratitude.

Gratitude Is Not a Bypass

Turning toward gratitude is not denial or avoidance of the painful parts of life; rather, it is noticing what else is present. You can experience difficulty and still appreciate what you have. Gratitude is always here. It is like the sun on an overcast day; although you can't see it, it is there. Gratitude is always within reach if you feed it. The Benedictine monk and author David Steindl-Rast wrote, "We are never more than one grateful thought away from peace of heart." With a peaceful heart, you can handle any challenge that comes your way.

Perhaps you can try feeding gratitude right now. After reading the next few sentences, put this book down and follow a few breaths. Then ask yourself, "In this moment, what is there in my life that I can be grateful for?" Start with what is most immediate, and expand from there. Once you spend a few moments feeding gratitude, see what you notice about your frame of mind and how you feel in your body.

Assuming you experienced gratitude, did you notice any shifts in your attitude or in how you feel in your body? These shifts can be subtle. If you could not generate feelings of gratitude or did not notice any shifts in your outlook or sensations, don't worry about it. It may take more effort for you to find something that evokes gratitude. Try again later under different circumstances.

Strengthening Your Gratitude Muscle

My wife and I have a daily gratitude practice that we do before we go to sleep at night. One of us will say to the other, "Share three things you are grateful for." Unless we are very tired, typically we mention more than three things, and there is often a story behind each thing mentioned. This also serves as a nice reminder of the day that has passed. I notice that when I travel on my own, I miss this practice. I also notice that the practice supports a deeper appreciation of what I experience throughout the day.

When you experience gratitude, you acknowledge your connection to the wider world that provides everything and holds your unique experience. Gratitude has a way of enhancing your satisfaction with life. As a caregiver you can use gratitude as a way to help the person you are caring for shift their outlook on their circumstances. You can help them achieve more peace. Brené Brown puts it this way: "I don't have to chase extraordinary moments to find happiness — it's right in front of me if I'm paying attention and practicing gratitude." You can help the person you care for pay attention to parts of their life that are beyond hardship or strain. You can try pointing them toward the light of gratitude. You might try in your own words, without expectation, something like, "I know you are struggling right now, but is there anything you feel grateful for?" This kind of inquiry may be difficult or even off-putting for some people. Their inability to express something that makes them feel grateful when you ask does not mean they will have nothing to share if you were to ask again on another day.

Gratitude Found in the Happiness of Others

If it is difficult to feel gratitude for something in our own life, we can still find gratitude when thinking about the happiness of others. In chapter 9 we touched on the Buddhist framework for cultivating an open heart known as the *brahmaviharas*, or the four heavenly abodes: compassion, kindness, equanimity, and appreciative or sympathetic joy. I believe the cultivation of any of these qualities supports the realization of the others. We have covered the first three of these in previous chapters, so let us now take a look at the fourth.

Appreciative joy is taking pleasure in the happiness or good fortune of others. It is recognizing that others' happiness contributes to our own happiness. It is the opposite of comparing ourselves to others or envying what others have that we do not. And, for most of us, it requires cultivation through practice.

There have been times when my activities and freedom have been extremely limited due to complications from the Crohn's disease I live with. During those times, I have thought about my wife and friends who are feeling good and enjoying themselves. I must admit that my thoughts would at times get stuck in what has been referred to as FOMO, or fear of missing out. Such fear is a close cousin of resentment. When I had the wherewithal to pause and observe my negative thinking, I was able to shift into appreciative joy by dropping into present-moment awareness. In direct experience of the present moment, my mind and heart are cleansed of comparing thoughts that feed envy. How awful the world would be if the joy and well-being of others stopped, just because I was feeling lousy or experiencing some difficulty. My more reflective self wants others to thrive and be happy. This is not some grand selfless ideal; it is a recognition of my expanded sense of self, my true self. The joy and well-being expressed by others is also my joy and well-being, and this feeds my gratitude.

Whether you foster gratitude by acknowledging what you have in your life or by taking joy in what others have, it will enhance your sense of well-being. Feeding gratitude may not come naturally, but by now I hope you have seen that making even a small effort to practice will yield big results in your well-being and happiness. When you experience gratitude and the happiness it produces, it is very likely that the person you care for, and others, will notice. And hopefully they will be able to find joy in seeing you happy and feel increased gratitude for your presence in their life.

[Practice]

You can try the gratitude practice at any point during your day. Even in the midst of struggling with a difficulty, you can shift your outlook by inviting gratitude into your mind and heart. This is a great way to end the day on a positive note before falling off to sleep.

- Settle your mind with a moment or two of following your breath. Keeping some of your attention on the breath, also notice your thoughts, emotions, and any obvious physical sensations.
- Ask yourself, "What do I have to feel grateful for in this moment?" Consider the people in your life, the food you enjoy, whatever comforts you have, and the natural features of the environment where you live. If you feel a lack of any of these things in your life, you might turn your thoughts to what you have experienced in the past.
- Take as long as you need to think about what you are grateful for. Once you find parts of your life that evoke gratitude, see if the experience changes how you feel in your body. Does gratitude impact your thoughts or emotions? Notice if anything shifts for you.
- Consider entering into your journal the things you are grateful for. You can refer back to your journal entry later if you find it difficult to access gratitude in the future.

CHAPTER 29

Calling On Our Teachers

May I hold in my heart and mind
The lessons learned from the caregivers
Who have gone before me
May I be inspired by expressions of kindness
I have witnessed

This chapter offers an invitation to recall people who supported you when you struggled through difficult times. Thinking of these people, you will be prompted to recall some of the qualities that made them skillful caregivers and positive role models. Through the lens of thinking about mentors and role models, you will be asked to consider how you may be inspiring others through your caregiving.

One of my favorite sessions we lead as part of our in-person Mindful Caregiving course is called "Imagining the Mindful Caregiver." This is an interactive session where participants recall two or three caregivers who either supported them or supported people close to them. Then we guide the participants to think about the lessons they learned from those caregivers. For most of the course participants, it is a joyful activity to recall those who extended love when care was needed.

I believe part of the usefulness of the session is reminding participants that they have mentors who have taught them lessons about caregiving. Many of us lack strong role models or genuine mentors. In the domain of popular culture, including social media, politics, sports, and entertainment, I see a dire shortage of healthy role models. Yet when we look at whom we have known in our own circle of friends, family and acquaintances, we can usually find mentors and role models.

The Dalai Lama reminds us of the essential role of the caring heart when he suggests, "Love and compassion are not luxuries, they are necessities. Without them, humanity would not survive." None of us would be here today without the support of others who made sacrifices for the sake of our health and well-being. Even if you were raised in an unhealthy or even abusive environment, there is likely someone who extended kindness and support to you.

Recalling Who Showed Up for You

When thinking about who supported you or showed up in times of need, it is useful to take a broad interpretation of the term *caregiver*. It is not necessary to restrict the category to those who provided care during illness. For instance, a teacher, coach, therapist, or spiritual leader could be considered a caregiver. Also, if you look beyond your personal life and consider people you have never actually met, such as someone from the public sphere, you may discover a role model or someone who inspires you.

I invite you to close your eyes and think about the times when you or someone close to you struggled with a challenge. Maybe it was a child or teenager trying to make sense of the world, or perhaps you or someone close to you faced a physical or mental health challenge. Did anyone offer support during these times of difficulty? If no struggles come to mind, perhaps someone showed up in a caring way when you or someone close to you was a child needing the support of an adult. Try to recall two or three people who displayed the qualities of positive caregiving. Notice how it feels as you think about them.

You might write down the names of these people in your journal, along with what you remember about how they showed up for you or someone close to you. When you think of them, what is it about their care that is notable for you? Can you name three qualities that you view as especially supportive in the care they provided? Are these qualities included in the care you provide? Perhaps they are qualities you would like to more fully express in your own caregiving. What gets in the way of expressing these qualities? What would it take for you to overcome whatever gets in your way?

Others Pay Attention to Your Caregiving

It is quite likely that the caregivers who demonstrated positive caregiving were not thinking about the impression they were making on you. Nonetheless, they did make an impression. As a caregiver, you probably do not provide care just because it may make a positive impression on others. However, I am confident that there are people in your life who take notice of the support you provide and learn valuable lessons from your example. You are very likely a caregiver role model to the people you know. Many qualities of your caregiving may inspire them if they ever find themselves in the role of caregiver.

Even if those around you are not thinking about what they might be learning from you, they still benefit from observing your caregiving. Recall the three beneficiaries of compassion we identified in chapter 15, including someone who witnesses an act of compassion. The person you are caring for is not the only one who benefits from your actions. The impact of your care ripples outward, and you never know who will benefit at some point.

Calling In Your Role Models

When caregiving becomes a struggle, you can call on your role models to inspire you to persevere and do your best. Whether these role models are living or deceased, they can continue to support you when you simply call them and their positive qualities to mind. You can invoke them as a source of warmth, care, and compassion. The usefulness of thinking about the role models you have witnessed is supported by a growing body of research. These studies, conducted by psychology researchers, have looked at the positive relationship between the use of compassion-associated imagery and the reduction of depression, stress, and anxiety.

You might even consider placing photos of your role models in a spot where you will see them regularly. Or you can use objects that are associated with these mentors as a reminder to call them in when needed. You can ask yourself what these teachers would say to you if they were present to witness your struggles. If they were with you, what would you want them to see in your attitude and actions related to caregiving?

When my mother was dying, I had this feeling that my role models were there with me and had my back. It was as if I could hear the voices of Frank, Eric, Irene, and others there with me when I did not know what to do or say, or was in deep despair. They were a profound source of comfort and confidence. Although they were not actually with me, I felt very supported.

You Are a Source of Inspiration

Who are the people who will someday feel your presence or support as they struggle to care for someone dear to them? If others are taking notice of your caregiving, what do you want them to see in the way you offer care? What lessons do you want them to take away from witnessing your caregiving?

You likely do the best you can in your role as caregiver, without worrying about who witnesses you. Of course, your caregiving will not always be an expression of your best self. As discussed in chapter 13, many things can get in the way of bringing your best self to your caregiving. Even when you feel you have fallen short, the way you recommit and come back to doing better will make an impression. The caregivers who have most inspired me are those who have been able to accept their human fallibility. Though they failed from time to time, they recognized the necessity of beginning again and trying to do better next time.

We should not expect our role models to be perfect. If all you see in them is perfection, perhaps they have not allowed their true self to be seen. I hope you show the people who are paying attention that shortcomings and even failure are a natural part of the caregiving experience — as is the recognition that each breath is an opportunity to begin again. Encouraging yourself to try again when you fall short is an act of kindness. By modeling kindness and vulnerability, you leave a lasting gift to those who follow you in the role of caregiver.

[Practice]

If you have not already done so, take some time to recall two or three caregivers who have modeled positive caregiving qualities. Write these names in your journal. Then write three positive qualities each caregiver demonstrated that you would like to embody more fully in your own caregiving. Circle the three qualities most important to you, and consider how you could more fully express these qualities in your caregiving. Also, consider what the obstacles are to expressing these qualities more fully. What would it take for you to overcome them?

Notice what emotions arise for you when you think of the caregivers who have inspired you. Try to hold on to any positive feelings.

CHAPTER 30

The Power of Intention

With each breath
With each thought and action
I move closer
To the one I am destined to become

You can choose to set intentions to address difficulties in your life or to evolve into the best possible caregiver you can become. This chapter discusses ways to use intention-setting in your caregiving and in life generally.

I find it remarkable that we human beings have the ability to think about the future and consider who we want to become later in life. It is important to plan for the future. It arrives faster than we expect. Thinking about the person we want to become in the future may seem contrary to cultivating and maintaining present-moment awareness. However, I find that considering my future self from time to time is very much about the present moment. What I do today has an effect on who I become tomorrow. With each thought, each action, each breath, I am practicing to become my future self. It does not happen by magic or by pretending to be that person. In fact, I must begin right where I am, in this moment, to evolve into the person I want to become.

In the Zen tradition, vows play an important role. I find that working with vows, or intentions, keeps us true to our best self. Vows, or intentions, are like the fletching on an arrow. The fletching provides stability to keep an arrow on course and assists with accuracy. Without it, an arrow will drift off course and miss its target. Even though we can see a target from where we are standing, we may need assistance to hit the bullseye as we move toward it. Vows help us hit the target.

Setting Intention with Vows

Each day, following my morning meditation, I recite the four great vows. The vows are chanted in Zen centers at various times throughout the day. I see these vows or precepts as a form of intention-setting. The vows offer clarity and remind me of who I want to be in the world. By reciting the four great vows, I strengthen my resolve. There are numerous translations, but I am fond of the four great vows recited at the Upaya Zen Center in Santa Fe, New Mexico.

> *Creations are numberless, I vow to free them.*
> *Delusions are inexhaustible, I vow to transform them.*
> *Reality is boundless, I vow to perceive it.*
> *The awakened way is unsurpassable, I vow to embody it.*

For me, these vows are about the existence of suffering and the possibility of alleviating it, both my own suffering and the suffering of others. While there are countless interpretations of their meaning, this is how the four great vows inspire me:

Creations are numberless, I vow to free them.

I intend to live a life of service to others. I try to do what I can to lessen the suffering of all beings when I witness it. This means showing up with compassion for others and myself. I cannot possibly do this 24/7, and I accept that. Also, I acknowledge that I cannot possibly address all the suffering in the world. I vow to do my best and extend kindness and compassion in all my waking hours.

Delusions are inexhaustible, I vow to transform them.

I intend to live my life without being overly attached to my way of interpreting the world around me. I do not want to automatically assume that what I think is happening around me is objective reality. This becomes especially important when I make assumptions regarding what I observe about others and what they are thinking or feeling. I want to catch myself when I project my own ideas or emotions onto someone else, believing the projection to be truth. I want to remember that my thoughts are only my thoughts and not necessarily facts. This vow reminds me to stay curious about what I observe and to ask more questions. I also know that to function in this world, there will be times when I need to trust my assumptions. This vow is primarily about my mind and my difficulties, but I also see it as a reminder that I can encourage others to question their assumptions as a way to alleviate their suffering.

Reality is boundless, I vow to perceive it.

I intend in each moment to be with things as they are. I see this as the flip side of the previous vow. As an expression of my curiosity, I want to investigate, through direct observation, the world around me. Staying true to my practice, I try in each moment to return to present-moment awareness by asking myself, *What is true in this moment?* I want to explore the world around me with an open mind, and I do this by dropping the filters that potentially cause biases in my thinking.

The awakened way is unsurpassable, I vow to embody it.

I intend to awaken in each moment by being aware of what is actually happening, both internally and in the world around me. I want to replace resistance to the encounters and activities in my life with present-moment awareness. I try to engage others in a way that makes them feel seen and important, even when the encounter is brief. I acknowledge that I will also get distracted by persistent thoughts, aches and pains, and negative emotions. However, I vow to remember that I can always return to embodying the awakened way.

The four great vows are relevant both to my moment-to-moment existence and to becoming the person I want to become. When I am nearing the end of my life and I look back on how I have lived, if I can honestly say that I did my best to live by these vows, I think I will be at peace with myself. Intentions and vows help prepare us for that future process of reckoning with our lives.

Perhaps you have observed that the great vows are contradictory in nature. There is something impossible about them. If something is numberless, how can it be freed? If inexhaustible, how can it be transformed? If boundless, can it be fully perceived? If unsurpassable, how can I possibly embody it? Impossible, yet I do my best to live in accordance with the vows. I try, knowing I will not succeed. This is humbling, and this is human.

I remember hearing Martha deBarros, one of the founders of Zen Hospice Project, talking about precepts as "rules that are meant to be broken." She was speaking to the fallibility of humans. The founder of Soto Zen, Dogen Zenji, said, "Hitting the mark is the result of ninety-nine failures." We take on vows, precepts, or intentions and we do our best, knowing we will fail. And, even though we fail, we still move toward the target of who we want to become.

Addressing Suffering with Intention

I learned, by engaging in and guiding initiation rites, that the only way to survive intense suffering is to have strong intentions. When I am guiding rites-of-passage programs, we spend as much time as needed working with each participant to clarify a succinct and strong intention for going out onto the land alone and forgoing food and comfort. We call this process *mirroring for intention.* I feel confident that a strong, clear intention will help keep a participant who is fasting safe. It will help them stay out when they are miserable and wanting nothing more than to call the whole thing off so they can come back to camp. Without a strong intention, they will not be able to hold themself accountable to their fellow participants and to their larger purpose. Their intention is different from our agreement that they will return to camp early if they are ever in danger.

I am grateful that I have the powerful tool of intention-setting to get through difficulties. Whenever I enter into a situation that I know will be challenging — a difficult conversation, a work meeting, or some other activity that may ask of me more than I think I can provide — I set an intention for myself. Sometimes the intention helps me deal with the situation, and sometimes I forget about my intention. But even when I forget about it, the setting of intention reminds me that all I need to do is try to do my best. In setting intentions, I find permission to just be human. This relieves some of the pressure that can contribute to resistance and uneasiness.

My wife and I enjoy walking outside first thing in the morning. We get outside to look at the sky and feel the warmth of the sun. It helps us wake up and, so we have been told, promotes better sleep. On these walks, we will often ask each other what our intention is for the day. Sharing our intentions reminds us that we have resources to draw upon when things get difficult. The intention can be as simple as "I intend to welcome whatever I encounter with an open heart and clear attention." Or "I intend to stay focused on what is in front of me."

Short-Term and Long-Term Intentions

These morning exchanges are focused on what I call short-term intentions, which are slightly different from long-term intentions. Short-term intention-setting will help you prepare to show up fully for events and activities you know you will encounter in the near future. These intentions are shaped by the type of event or activity you expect to engage in.

Before I visit my father, I set an intention so I don't lose sight of the need to also take care of myself. I try to do certain things to stay physically and emotionally healthy when I enter his home. As my wife is fond of saying, the intentions I establish "set me up for a win." Perhaps there is something in particular that I want to discuss with him while I am visiting, and the intention helps keep me focused on the conversation so I do not miss the opportunity before needing to return home.

Long-term intentions are typically more general and focused on who you want to become. When we send fasters out, knowing they will encounter intense suffering, the intention we uncover with them is longer term. A lot is at stake with this sort of intention, so it has a greater influence on behavior. An example of this type of intention might be, "I am an elder who inspires those around me by my actions. May all my actions express my open heart and my commitment to family." Or "I am a man who recognizes his strengths and his weaknesses. May I give away my unique gifts to the world, through every action and every encounter."

The values affirmation practice you did in chapter 15 is a very useful exercise to help clarify a larger purpose in your caregiving and in your life. If you feel inspired to think about a longer-term intention or vow, you might revisit this practice activity. This will give you a framework for thinking about what matters most to you as you think about who you are becoming.

The most powerful intentions are short, direct, and easy to remember. An intention of one or two sentences is ideal. The shorter the intention, the easier it will be to remember. I find it useful to begin an intention with "I intend to..." Or you might begin with a "May I..." statement: "May I keep part of my attention on my breath when I feel mistreated." Or "May I feel my feet on the ground when there is chaotic activity around me." Another possible form is "Let me..." as in, "Let me remember to be kind to myself when I feel overwhelmed."

Using Intention-Setting in Your Caregiving

As a caregiver, you can use intention to guide you in becoming the best possible caregiver you can be. Regardless of the type of caregiving you do and of whether or not you think you had a choice in becoming a caregiver, one day you will no longer be in the role. When you look back at the experience, what do you want to remember? How will you want to feel about the way you showed up in the role?

The practice activity for this chapter will guide you in the process of setting an intention. Though it is a simple practice, it can have a big impact on the care you provide. While the practice activity is focused on a particular event or activity, it will prepare you to step back and consider your larger purpose as a caregiver and set a longer-term intention for evolving into that person. Let the practice of setting an intention guide you to become a caregiver you will be happy and proud to remember.

[Practice]

- Take a moment to think about a future event or activity you will participate in. This may or may not be related to your caregiving role. Perhaps it is an activity that feels intimidating or causes stress.
- Whatever the event or activity, think about a short intention for how you want to show up for the experience. Who do you want to be in the event or activity? Try using the "May I..." form to craft your intention.
- Write down your intention. Remember to keep it succinct, a sentence or two, or three at the most, so you can easily remember it.
- Consider sharing your intention with someone you trust so they can be your witness. Or you can post it somewhere in your home where you will see it. Keeping the intention close will help you remember it at the time of the event.

After the event, think about your intention and if you lived up to it. If you forgot about your intention or if it made no difference in how you behaved or felt, it's no big deal. You will have another opportunity to set an intention. You always have the option to step back and think about how you show up for the caregiving you offer.

Conclusion

With each ending
A new beginning unfolds before me
May I have the courage to meet fully
Whatever comes next

It has been an honor to share with you ideas and practices that have decreased suffering in my own life. In concluding this book, I hope that you never underestimate your resilience or the potential you have as a caregiver to change a life and the world. Our world and your community, filled with so much suffering, need you. When your efforts feel insignificant, when you are exhausted, please remember that your actions and your sacrifices make a difference.

I will end with a passage from the late Tibetan Buddhist teacher Tulku Thondup Rinpoche. For many years, this beautiful teaching has been a source of inspiration to me. These wise words remind me that even through struggles, caring for others is not only a noble and generous endeavor but also a path toward growth and well-being. May your experience as a caregiver be gentle and a source of joy and deep purpose in your life.

Taking care of someone will become a meditation for you, a practice.
Meditation, as you know, creates many good merits.
It may not be visible to others, but our helping each other is
a merit-making process.
If you need to help someone, you will be practicing the six perfections
(patience, generosity, discipline, diligence, contemplation, and wisdom).

This is the most important practice.
Even giving a mouthful of food could include all these perfections.
Maybe some hardship will be involved, but then you cultivate patience…
Whatever you do to help, do it with total concentration.
The wisdom in this case would be the wisdom of non-self, giving as a dedication, as a service to others, with no attachment or grasping.
Do whatever you do joyfully, because discipline — the true meaning of the word — is characterized by doing something with joy.
Even the little things: see them as an opportunity, a blessing, a meditation, as spiritual practice.
Then, even if it's difficult, it will be good.
If you use hardships in a proper way, they can even bring inner peace.

Acknowledgments

I want to express my gratitude to those who supported me in writing this book. My beloved Kristin has been my ultimate champion and reader. Without her in my life, many things would not get done. I have been blessed to have many friends who have offered encouragement and useful feedback. A big thank-you to my colleagues at Zen Caregiving Project: Mary Doane, Alistair Shanks, Sarah Bain, and Chris Panos, who have worked with me over the years to create an impactful program to support caregivers. I have had wonderful teachers who have modeled mindful compassionate care: Frank Ostaseski, Eric Poché, Irene Smith, Tova Green, and BJ Miller, to name just a few. Jason Gardner and the team at New World Library immediately understood the relevance of this book and have been big advocates. I have felt immense support from the Mesa Refuge staff and from Alice Dorrance, who made it possible for me to dedicate two uninterrupted weeks to work on my manuscript in a stunningly beautiful and inspiring place. I am eternally grateful to the many people living with serious illness who welcomed me into their life to receive care and companionship. Finally, a deep bow of gratitude to all who are quoted in this book; your dedication to helping others was a deep source of inspiration that at times kept me going.

Notes

Chapter 1: Why Mindfulness

p. 11 *According to the American Mindfulness Research Association:* American Mindfulness Research Association, "'Mindfulness' in Academic Journal Article Titles by Year: 1980–2024," https://goamra.org/Library.

p. 12 *The study found that the four-week online:* Michael Juberg et al., "Investigating the Feasibility and Effects of an Online Mindfulness Family Caregiver Training Program," *Mindfulness* 14 (2023): 1531–41, https://doi.org/10.1007/s12671-023-02126-3.

Chapter 2: This Perfect Moment

p. 19 *A study conducted in India in 2015:* Badri Bajaj and Neerja Pande, "Mediating Role of Resilience in the Impact of Mindfulness on Life Satisfaction and Affect as Indices of Subjective Well-Being," *Personality and Individual Differences* 93 (2016): 63–67, https://doi.org/10.1016/j.paid.2015.09.005.

Chapter 5: Working Skillfully with Big Emotions

p. 38 *The American Psychological Association defines emotions: American Psychological Association*, "Emotions," accessed March 23, 2024, apa.org/topics/emotions.

Chapter 6: Modeling Presence

p. 45 *Martha was everything good and right:* Richard Rohr, *The Naked Now: Learning to See as the Mystics See* (Crossroads Publishing, 2009), 58.

p. 49 *Jane Verity, the founder of Dementia Care International:* Jane Verity, "Spark of Life 5 Core Emotional Needs," *Dementia Care International*, May 8, 2009, dementiacareinternational .com/2009/05/spark-of-life-5-core-emotional-needs-2/.

Chapter 7: Mindful Communication

p. 55 *Sociologist and psychologist Sherry Turkle:* Sherry Turkle, *Reclaiming Conversation: The Power of Talk in a Digital Age* (Penguin, 2015), 20–22.

p. 58 *"In the beginner's mind, there are many possibilities":* Shunryu Suzuki, *Zen Mind, Beginner's Mind* (Weatherhill, 1970), 21.

Chapter 10: Becoming a Compassionate Companion

p. 82 "*Injustice anywhere is a threat to justice everywhere":* Martin Luther King, *Letter from a Birmingham Jail* (Birmingham, AL: April 16, 1962).

Chapter 11: Loving-Kindness

p. 89 *The study found that a regular practice of loving-kindness:* Barbara L. Fredrickson at al., "Open Hearts Build Lives: Positive Emotions, Induced through Loving-Kindness Meditation, Build Consequential Personal Resources, *Journal of Personality and Social Psychology* 95, no. 5 (November 2008):1045–62.

p. 89 *Other studies have found similar results:* Xianglong Zeng et al., "The Effect of Loving-Kindness Meditation on Positive Emotions: A Meta-Analytic Review," *Frontiers in Psychology*, November 2, 2015, https://doi.org/10.3389/fpsyg.2015.01693.

p. 89 *Take for example the various necessities of our life:* Thupten Jinpa, *A Fearless Heart: How the Courage to Be Compassionate Can Transform Our Lives* (Avery, 2015), 164–65.

Chapter 12: Self-Compassion

p. 92 *"If your compassion does not include yourself":* Jack Kornfield, *Buddha's Little Instruction Book* (Bantam, 1994), 28.

p. 95 *Research shows that people with higher levels of self-compassion:*

Kristin Neff, *Self-Compassion: The Proven Power of Being Kind to Yourself* (William Morrow, 2011), 94.

Chapter 13: Barriers to Compassion

p. 102 *Psychologist and researcher Susan Fiske:* Susan Fiske and Shelley Taylor, "Social Cognition," in *Handbook of Social Psychology*, ed. Gardner Lindzey and Elliot Aronson (Random House, 1985), 151–92.

p. 110 *"While empathy refers to our general capacity to resonate":* Tania Singer and Olga M. Klimecki, "Empathy and Compassion," *Current Biology* 24, no. 18 (2014): R875–R878, https://doi.org/10.1016/j.cub.2014.06.054.

p. 112 *People who act to address the needs of others:* Emma Seppälä, "Compassionate Mind, Healthy Body," *Greater Good Magazine*, July 24, 2013, https://greatergood.berkeley.edu/article/item/compassionate_mind_healthy_body.

Chapter 14: Overcoming Barriers to Compassion

p. 116 *We learn to unhook our awareness from the restless:* Thupten Jinpa, *A Fearless Heart: How the Courage to Be Compassionate Can Transform Our Lives* (Avery, 2015), 111.

Chapter 15: Compassion Is Contagious

p. 127 *"a positive emotional state that is described as feeling inspired":* Jonathan Haidt, "Elevation and the Positive Psychology of Morality," in *Flourishing: Positive Psychology and the Life Well-Lived*, ed. Corey L. M. Keyes and Jonathan Haidt (American Psychological Association, 2003), 275–89.

p. 127 *"positive emotions may loosen the hold":* Barbara L. Fredrickson, "Cultivating Positive Emotions to Optimize Health and Well-Being," *Prevention & Treatment* 3, Article 0001a (March 7, 2000), https://doi.org/10.1037/1522-3736.3.1.31a.

p. 129 *"sometimes it is necessary to reteach a thing":* Galway Kinnell, *Selected Poems* (Houghton Mifflin,1982), 126.

Chapter 16: The Ever-Present Nature of Loss

p. 136 *"Loss has already transfigured your life":* Jeff Foster, "You Will Lose Everything," *Life Without a Centre* (website), accessed October 17, 2025.

p. 136 *Eight out of ten family caregivers report:* Laura Skufca and Chuck Rainville, "Caregiving Can Be Costly — Even Financially," *Caregiving Out-of-Pocket Costs Study 2021* (AARP, June 2021), https://doi.org/10.26419/res.00473.001.

p. 138 *Twenty-three percent of caregivers in the US report: AARP 2020 Report: Caregiving in the U.S.* (AARP, May 2020), https://doi.org/10.26419/ppi.00103.001.

Chapter 18: A Mindfulness-Based Approach to Grief

p. 151 "*To honor our grief, to grant it space":* Francis Weller, *The Wild Edge of Sorrow: Rituals of Renewal and the Sacred Work of Grief* (North Atlantic, 2015), xxiii.

Chapter 19: Supporting Others with Their Loss

p. 157 "*We're always dying to things":* Anthony De Mello, *Awareness: A De Mello Spirituality Conference in His Own Words* (Image, 1992), 151.

Chapter 20: Inviting Conversations About Loss

p. 172 *"Hope almost always makes sure that it is too late":* Stephen Jenkinson, *Die Wise: A Manifesto for Sanity and Soul* (North Atlantic Books, 2015), 134.

Chapter 22: Preparing for the Dying Phase

p. 187 *"Love is watching someone die":* Death Cab for Cutie, "What Sarah Said," on *Plans* (Atlantic Records, 2005), CD.

p. 188 *"I move from one moment to the next new moment":* Kim Addonizio, "Living with the Dying: An Interview with Frank Ostaseski," *The Sun*, no. 165 (August 1989), https://www.thesunmagazine.org/publications/3/editions/2115.

p. 190 *In the period between 2000 and 2020:* Center to Advance Palliative Care, *Growth of Palliative Care in US Hospitals: 2022 Snapshot (2000–2020)*, https://www.capc.org/documents/1031/?clickthrough_doc_id=core.cmsdocument.

p. 192 *It depends on the type of illness:* Stephen R. Connor et al., "Comparing Hospice and Nonhospice Patient Survival among Patients Who Die within a Three-Year Window," *Journal of Pain Symptom Management* 33, no. 3. (March 2007): 238–46, doi:10.1016/j.jpainsymman.2006.10.010.

Chapter 25: Working with Storied Self and Essential Self

p. 223 *"The essential self is what allows us to relate":* Marguerite Manteau-Rao, *Caring for a Loved One with Dementia: A Mindfulness-Based Guide for Reducing Stress and Making the Best of Your Journey Together* (New Harbinger, 2016), 185.

Chapter 26: Sharing Your Story

p. 228 *"What is the source of our first suffering?":* Gaston Bachelard, trans. Maria Jolas, *The Poetics of Reverie: Childhood, Language, and the Cosmos* (Beacon, 1994), 15.

p. 230 *Gigi Coyle and Jack Zimmerman established:* Jack Zimmerman with Virginia Coyle, *The Way of Council* (Bramble Books, 1996), 28–38.

p. 232 *"We are important and our lives are important":* Natalie Goldberg, *Writing Down the Bones: Freeing the Writer Within* (Shambhala, 2005), 43.

Chapter 27: Healing Touch

p. 238 *"There is strong evidence that many older adults":* Clifford Singer, "Health Effects of Social Isolation and Loneliness," *Journal of Aging Life Care* 28, no. 1 (Spring 2018): 4–8.

Chapter 28: Feeding Gratitude

p. 243 *"It is difficult to say thank you":* Zenju Earthlyn Manuel, *The Shamanic Bones of Zen: Revealing the Ancestral Spirit and Mystical Heart of a Sacred Tradition* (Shambhala, 2022), 148.

p. 244 *"We are never more than one grateful thought away":* David Steindl-Rast, *Essential Writings* (Orbis Books, 2010), 65.

p. 245 *"I don't have to chase extraordinary moments":* Brené Brown, *Daring Greatly: How the Courage to Be Vulnerable Transforms the Way We Live, Love, Parent, and Lead* (Avery, 2015), 41.

Chapter 29: Calling On Our Teachers

p. 249 *"Love and compassion are not luxuries":* Dalai Lama XIV and Howard C. Cutler, *The Art of Happiness: A Handbook for Living* (Riverhead Books, 1998), 19.

p. 251 *These studies, conducted by psychology researchers:* Kirsten McEwan and Paul Gilbert, "A Pilot Feasibility Study Exploring the Practising of Compassionate Imagery Exercises in a Nonclinical Population," *Psychology Psychotherapy* 89, no. 2 (June 2016):239–43, https://doi.org/10.1111/papt.12078.

Caregiver Resources

Advanced Medical Directives

Five Wishes: fivewishes.org

The Conversation Project: theconversationproject.org

Advance Health Care Directive Form: Free advance health care directive forms by state from AARP: https://www.aarp.org/caregiving/financial-legal/free-printable-advance-directives/.

POLST form: Almost all states have their own POLST form. Please request a POLST form from your health provider. Visit polst.org for the latest information on establishing a nationally recognized POLST form.

Prepare: prepareforyourcare.org/en/prepare/welcome

Advocacy

Caring Across Generations: caringacross.org

National Domestic Workers Alliance: domesticworkers.org

Care Can't Wait: carecantwait.org

Administration for Community Living National Strategy to Support Family Caregivers: acl.gov/CaregiverStrategy

Moving Forward: movingforwardcoalition.org

Compassion, Self-Compassion

Center for Mindful Self-Compassion: centerformsc.org

Dr. Kristin Neff: self-compassion.org

Compassion Institute: compassioninstitute.com

Center for Compassion and Altruism Research and Education: ccare.stanford.edu
Compassionate Mind Foundation: compassionatemind.co.uk
Charter for Compassion: charterforcompassion.org

Death and Dying/Palliative Care

Compassion & Choices: compassionandchoices.org
National Hospice and Palliative Care Organization(NHPCO): nhpco.org
Mettle Health: mettlehealth.com

Dementia Care

Alzheimer's Association: alz.org
Lorenzo's House: lorenzoshouse.org
Presence Care Project: presencecareproject.com

Family Caregiving

Zen Caregiving Project: zencaregiving.org
Commonweal: commonweal.org
Family Caregiver Alliance: caregiver.org
Rosalynn Carter Institute for Caregivers: rosalynncarter.org

Grief Support

Evermore: evermore.org
Grief.com: grief.com
End Well Project: endwellproject.org
Death Over Dinner: deathoverdinner.org
Death Cafe: deathcafe.com
The Dinner Party: thedinnerparty.org
Reimagine: letsreimagine.org

Inspiration

Grateful Living: grateful.org
Good News Network: goodnewsnetwork.org
Greater Good Science Center: ggsc.berkeley.edu

Zen/Mindfulness/Meditation Practice

San Francisco Zen Center: sfzc.org
Upaya Zen Center: upaya.org
Mindful: mindful.org
American Mindfulness Research Association: goamra.org
Jon Kabat-Zinn: jonkabat-zinn.com
Spirit Rock: spiritrock.org
UC San Diego Center for Mindfulness: cih.ucsd.edu/mindfulness
AudioDharma: audiodharma.org

About the Author

Roy Remer is the executive director of Zen Caregiving Project in San Francisco, California. In 1997 he trained with Zen Hospice Project (ZHP) to become a volunteer and served at the bedside for six years at the guest house facility before serving for seven years on San Francisco's Laguna Honda Hospital's palliative care ward. Roy served on the ZHP board of directors from 2002 until 2008. In 2008 he completed a yearlong end-of-life caregiver training at the Metta Institute in Sausalito, California. Roy has been developing curriculum and teaching Mindful Caregiving Education courses since 2015.

A dedicated practitioner in the Soto Zen lineage, Roy is a student at the San Francisco Zen Center. He is certified by the Stanford University School of Medicine Center for Compassion and Altruism Research and Education (CCARE) and the Compassion Institute as a Compassion Cultivation Training (CCT©) instructor. Roy serves on the board of directors of Enso Village, a Zen-inspired senior living community in Healdsburg, California.

Roy also guides wilderness-based rites-of-passage programs in partnership with EarthWays LLC of Sebastopol, California.

For more information about Roy and Zen Caregiving Project's courses and workshops, please visit zencaregiving.org.

NEW WORLD LIBRARY is dedicated to publishing books and other media that inspire and challenge us to improve the quality of our lives and the world.

We are a socially and environmentally aware company. We recognize that we have an ethical responsibility to our readers, our authors, our staff members, and our planet.

We serve our readers by creating the finest publications possible on personal growth, creativity, spirituality, wellness, and other areas of emerging importance. We serve our authors by working with them to produce and promote quality books that reach a wide audience. We serve New World Library employees with generous benefits, significant profit sharing, and constant encouragement to pursue their most expansive dreams.

We print our books with soy-based ink on paper from sustainably managed forests. We power our Northern California office with solar energy, and we respectfully acknowledge that it is located on the ancestral lands of the Coast Miwok Indians. We also contribute to nonprofit organizations working to make the world a better place for us all.

Our products are available wherever books are sold.

customerservice@NewWorldLibrary.com
Phone: 415-884-2100 or 800-972-6657
Orders: Ext. 110
Fax: 415-884-2199
NewWorldLibrary.com